Smoking, Health & Personality

Smoking, Health & Personality

H.J. Eysenck

With a new foreword by
Stuart Brody

Routledge
Taylor & Francis Group
LONDON AND NEW YORK

Originally published in 1965 by Cox and Wyman, Ltd.

First published 2000 by Transaction Publishers

2 Park Square, Milton Park, Abingdon, Oxfordshire OX14 4RN
711 Third Avenue, New York, NY 10017

Routledge is an imprint of the Taylor & Francis Group, an informa business

First issued in hardback 2018

Library of Congress Catalog Number: 99-087782

Library of Congress Cataloging-in-Publication Data

Eysenck, H. J. (Hans Jurgen), 1916-
Smoking, health and personality / by H. J. Eysenck ; with a new foreword by Stuart Brody.
p. cm.
Originally published: 1965.
Includes bibliographical references and index.
ISBN 0-7658-0639-8 (paper : alk. paper)
1. Tobacco—Physiological effect. 2. Smoking—Psychological aspects. I. Title.

RA1242. T6 E9 2000
616.86'5—dc21 99-087782

ISBN 13: 978-0-7658-0639-0 (pbk)
ISBN 13: 978-1-138-53263-2 (hbk)

Contents

Illustrations

I do not reject the use of statistics, but I condemn not trying to go beyond them.

CLAUDE BERNARD

Foreword

IN THIS BOOK, H.J. Eysenck does more than critically review the literature, present longitudinal studies showing that psychological characteristics are far more potent predictors of heart disease and cancer than smoking behavior, and demonstrate that psychological treatment can halve death rates (unlike massive campaigns which exhort people to eschew tobacco or cholesterol and which have little or no demonstrable health benefits). He also speaks the unspeakable, iconoclastically attacking the cherished attribution of millions of deaths to smoking.

At the time of my writing this foreword, American attorneys are reaping the billion dollar benefits of a legal form of extortion of the tobacco companies, in which it is alleged that the defendants are responsible for excess health costs of the indigent. Besides the attorneys' donations to the Democratic Party, there is also a noteworthy financial connection between the National Cancer Institute and nominal charities such as the American Cancer Society, in which political coalitions were built with taxpayer money (detailed in Cancerscam, by Bennett & DiLorenzo). Researchers' funding and fame are also largely contingent on following the party line. Compared to some of these influential forces, the tobacco companies are nearly free of venality.

However, money is not the only reason people wage wars. Just as religion, clan, and nationalism may have led to more deaths than avarice did, so too is the defense of an ideology a basis for an assault on science. Slaying Goliath corporations appeals to some, as does the notion that if not for some external impediment, we could indefinitely delay the ultimate sadness. The external aspect deserves comment: it avoids the awareness that much of the devil is within, in our genes and our personalities.

As I described in a different context in my book (*Sex at Risk: Lifetime Number of Partners, Frequency of Intercourse, and the*

Low AIDS Risk of Vaginal Intercourse), risk-factor epidemiology has been manipulated for political purposes. Smokers tend to differ from nonsmokers in several important ways (personality features that lead to suboptimal self-regulation, less education, lower income, poorer diets, more recreational drug use, etc.). A failure to fully adjust for these differences leads to all of the blame being heaped on smoking.

Not surprisingly, after its first publication, *Smoking, Health, and Personality*, was the subject of vitriolic attacks, and Eysenck was accused (among other things) of obtaining "impossible" results. His work was conveniently omitted from many subsequent discussions of the topic (the bibliographic analog of Eysenck having been physically prevented from speaking on intelligence research at some universities). However, other recently published longitudinal studies have also found that personality is the best predictor of longevity. Friedman and colleagues, using data from a several decade longitudinal study initiated by Terman, found that even considering the effects of smoking and drinking alcohol, the personality trait of conscientiousness was the best predictor (other than the sex of the subject) of survival. Seltzer commented on the lack of relationship between smoking and coronary disease in the Framingham study when personality characteristics were included as a confounding variable, and how political pressure led to the suppression of this information. These studies, like some others of depression predicting subsequent morbidity and mortality, used broader personality measures than those used by Eysenck in this book, resulting in smaller effect sizes.

When I met with Eysenck in August 1996, he appeared a bit frail, but active and with a continuing sense of mission. He indicated his desire that the studies in this volume be replicated. Unfortunately, this was not possible during his lifetime. This book is an important part of his very large scholarly legacy, one to be prized as much for its sense of scientific curiosity and libertarianism as for its data.

Stuart Brody, PhD
Adjunct Research Professor of Medical Psychology
University of Tübingen

Introduction

Tobacco, divine, rare, superexcellent tobacco, which goes far beyond all their panaceas, potable gold and philosopher's stones, a sovereign remedy to all diseases. . . . But, as it is commonly abused by most men, which take it as tinkers do ale, 'tis a plague, a mischief, a violent purger of goods, lands, health, hellish, devilish and damned tobacco, the ruin and overthrow of body and soul.

RICHARD BURTON

MY LOVE-HATE relationship with the cigarette began a long time ago. I was thirteen at the time and I can well remember how I rather truculently told my grandmother, who was taking care of me, that I wanted to start smoking. I don't know what kind of a reaction I expected to get from her but she simply gave me sixpence and sent me down to the corner store to buy some cigarettes. When I had done that she calmly showed me how to light one and how to smoke it. Then she left me to it. I had a vague feeling that this was not quite the right thing to do; somehow it seemed to take all the fun out of it. I did persevere for a few days but finally decided that there was not much amusement to be got out of it and gave it up. I am sure if she had made a fuss, forbidden me to smoke and threatened to tell my father, the whole thing would have been much more amusing, and I might even have continued. However, in spite of a few sporadic attempts during the next few months smoking just didn't seem to fill any of my needs, and I decided to rather turn to wine, women and song. Unfortunately, I had a voice like a tone-deaf crow and I hated the taste of alcohol even more than that of nicotine; apart from these drawbacks the programme suited me fine, and I never returned to cigarettes until a few years later when I had a little disagreement on political matters with Adolph Hitler and became a refugee. I also became an impecunious student, and the combination of stresses was sufficient to make me try cigarettes again. This time, I must have been ripe for whatever smoking had to offer, because I took it up seriously and only poverty and later the rationing system during the War kept my consumption down to a rather moderate amount.

When the War was over I began to smoke more and more until finally I took up a visiting professorship at the University of Philadelphia on the Eastern Seaboard of the United States. The high pay and the low price of American cigarettes combined to make me go up into the two-packets-a-day class and I began to suffer from some of the consequences of smoking so much. I soon got short of breath when playing tennis; I started coughing early in the morning and cigarettes just didn't seem to taste of anything any more. In other words, I had become a true slave of the habit. When I returned to England in 1950 the Chancellor of the Exchequor had just turned the screw a little more and increased duty on tobacco to a quite unreasonable amount, or so it seemed to me. This, combined with all the ills of which I was complaining, set me to thinking that it was really absurd for a psychologist who prided himself on being an expert on the creation and extinction of habits to be subject to habit himself, and apparently find difficulties in breaking the habit. Smoking for pleasure was one thing but smoking, although you didn't get any more fun out of it, and simply because it had become an unbreakable habit, that was quite another. I decided there and then to give it up and have never smoked another cigarette since.

Fortunately, all this happened before the great controversy about smoking and lung cancer burst upon the medical world and later on made the headlines and put many smokers into a very unenviable position. Should they go on smoking and run the risk of suffering a very painful and lingering death of lung cancer or should they give up smoking and deprive themselves of a solace and a pleasure which they valued extremely highly? I was very pleased not to be faced with this dilemma, but I have always felt extremely sorry for those who are still left to make up their minds.

In the next few years, I heard and read reports of the work done by R. Doll and A. B. Hill on the relationship between smoking and cancer of the lung, but my first real encounter with the problem occurred when I was travelling from the International Congress of Psychology in Montreal, where I had been reading a paper on my theory of personality, to San Francisco, where I was taking up a teaching appointment at the University of California at Berkeley. In the same compartment as myself was a well-known and respected physician about 55 years of age who was travelling to a medical convention in San Francisco. He was just reading a paper by E. C. Hammond and D. Horn which appeared in the *Journal of the American Medical Association* and in which they reported the results of a follow-up study of 187,766 men, relating their smoking habits and death rates. He was a very heavy cigarette smoker indeed and the careful work and excellent logic of these two investigators had impressed him deeply. I told him of some of the criticisms that had been made of the English work, which also applied to the American study, and in particular I told him of the hypothesis put forward by Sir Ronald Fisher, the famous statistician and geneticist, that some of the relationship, if not all, between smoking and lung cancer might be due to genetic causes, the same persons being predisposed to smoke and to contract lung cancer. While he admitted the force of these arguments he nevertheless complained with a rather wry smile that it didn't really matter to him whether he died of lung cancer because he smoked cigarettes or because he was predisposed genetically; what he wanted to avoid was dying of lung cancer altogether! I admitted that he had a point there and we left the argument in this rather inconclusive state.

At Berkeley I had a lot of time to think about this problem and it linked up with the course of lectures on personality which I was giving at the time. Fisher had not actually proposed a theory as much as thrown out a hint of what a possible theory of the genetic determination of lung cancer might be like. Would it not be possible to link this up in some way with my own theory of personality, and thus make it possible to test the general hypothesis in question? I spent many evenings sitting in front of my bungalow, looking across the bay at the twinkling lights of San Francisco, trying to see how a testable theory might be put together from these various hints and notions. The problem, and it is really quite an intractable one, is essentially this. If some people are genetically predisposed to develop cancer then they must form a rather special group. The theory would only work if the same group was also predisposed to develop a desire for cigarette smoking in the course of their lives. This in turn means that people who smoke form a rather unusual group with certain characteristics, and it should be possible to detect what these characteristics might be. The hypothesis I was trying to work out was that the characteristics one would look for would be personality traits of one kind or another, and the problem was to find out just what these traits were. Many people had tried this, and there is a large literature on this subject, but most of them had done it on a fairly random basis. Instead of starting with a definite theory which could be supported or disproved, they had simply taken whatever came to hand in the way of tests or measures, and had applied these to usually rather odd, small and unusual groups of people. The results, as one might have expected, were very divergent; there was little agreement, and it was very difficult indeed to make any sense out of all this work. In the end I managed to come up with a theory which seemed at least worthy of further investigation, and when I returned to London I was able to carry out certain studies which gave confirmation to the main points of this theory.

In brief, I suggested that people of an extraverted type of personality would be more likely to smoke cigarettes than would more introverted people. If Fisher was right then it would also seem to follow from this that, unlikely as it might seem at first sight, extraverted people would be more prone to suffer from lung cancer than would introverts. The theory therefore would be that lung cancer and smoking are related, not because smoking causes lung cancer, but because the same people predisposed genetically to develop lung cancer were also predisposed genetically to take up smoking. This is the theory which I developed during those balmy days in California, and it is with this theory and the experiments conducted in relation to it that this book is concerned. I will not now discuss whether it helps the heavy smoker to decide the momentous question 'to smoke or not to smoke'; I will leave this to the last chapter. Nor do I want to discuss now whether the orthodox theory which considers smoking to be a causal factor in lung cancer is in fact wrong. These and many other questions I will try to answer after I have considered the evidence.

This book is concerned then with the relationships between three variables: smoking, disease, particularly lung cancer and coronary thrombosis, and personality. All the evidence to be considered is circumstantial; there is no direct evidence which does not rely on statistical investigation and logical interpretations. These are difficult matters and it is very easy to go wrong. As Dr R. Doll, himself one of the scientists most prominently associated with the promulgation of the theory that smoking causes cancer, has pointed out: 'When the nature of the disease makes it impossible to carry out logically conclusive experiments there is always room for honest difference of opinion. In the case of smoking it is particularly hard to envisage how a conclusive experiment could be carried out and no such experiments have been made.' Doll goes on to quote a famous saying of Claude Bernard, to the effect that 'There are no false theories and true theories, but only fertile theories and sterile theories.' It is my hope that the theory here proposed will not be a sterile one, but lead to further work which will ultimately ensure that the terrifying toll which lung cancer takes of human life and happiness will be reduced to more manageable proportions.

Chapter 1

The Origin and Growth of a Habit

What a blessing this smoking is! perhaps the greatest that we owe to the discovery of America.

SIR ARTHUR HELPS

AS BEFITS THE subject, the origin of the smoking habit appears shrouded in the myths of history. Archaeological work in Mexico has suggested that the tobacco plant played a great part in religious ceremonies among the Mayans before the beginning of our era. Over five hundred years ago the habit spread over the whole of Mexico and to the Red Indians and the South American Indians as well. Tobacco was consumed in various ways by smoking, chewing and as snuff; smoking was done not only by means of pipes and cigars but also by means of paper tubes some 3 or 4 inches in length known as *cigarros* or *papelitos*; these as well as the cigars and cigarettes which later became fashionable in Europe had a much greater nicotine content than do the smokes of our own time, and it seems miraculous that any human being could have been attracted to such very powerful drugs.

The discovery of America by Columbus in 1492 marks the beginning of the gradual subjugation of Europe to the tobacco plant. The form this conquest has taken has often been determined by rather curious circumstances. Thus in France, where tobacco was introduced in the second half of the sixteenth century, tobacco was not smoked but taken as snuff. The reason appears to be that Nicot, who was French Ambassador at the Portuguese court from 1559 to 1561, had sent some tobacco to

Catherine de Medici as a remedy for headaches to which her two sons were very prone. He sent the tobacco in the form of snuff; the habit spread, and smoking did not become popular until the reign of Louis XIV. The Spaniards, on the other hand, took to smoking cigars probably because Luis de Torres and Rodrigo de Perez, who had sailed with Columbus on his first expedition, explored the island of Cuba where they found the inhabitants smoking rolled leaves of tobacco.

The English of course took to pipe smoking rather than to snuff or to cigars. This was probably due to the fact that Drake on his return to England from Virginia in 1586 took with him some colonists who had adopted the habit of smoking tobacco through pipes from the Red Indians, whose 'pipe of peace' has become famous through many Western tales and television programmes. Raleigh himself took up the habit and introduced it to the court, and very soon men and women of all classes and ages could be found to smoke tobacco in the newfangled pipes.

Cigarette smoking, which is nowadays probably far more popular than all other forms of tobacco consumption combined, is of relatively recent origin in Europe and America, although as long ago as the middle of the eighteenth century many *papelitos* were smoked in Mexico City, not only by men but also by women. The first Europeans to be attracted to this habit were the Russians; they were followed by the French and English who made contact with the habit during the Crimean War. Americans took up the fashion even more slowly. As one might have expected they mechanized the manufacture of cigarettes in a way which made it possible for the first time to supply all the demands that might be made, and before the First World War there were in existence cigarette machines which could produce as many as 600 a minute; modern machines produce as many as 2,000,000 cigarettes a day. There were also great advances in the agricultural methods used for producing the plant and new ways of curing it were discovered. The scene was set for a gigantic leap forward and the past fifty years have shown a tremendous growth in the consumption of cigarettes as well as a corresponding decline in the use of other forms of tobacco.[1]

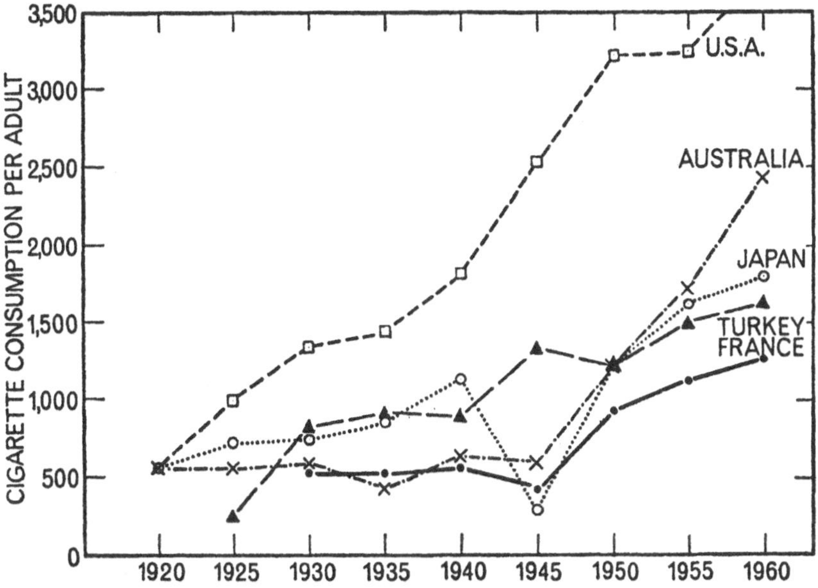

Fig. 1. Increase in cigarette consumption per adult in five countries from 1920–60. (Figures for some of the early years are not available for France and Turkey.) It is this increase in cigarette consumption which is held responsible for the increase in lung cancer by many people. As there is supposed to be a 20-year lag before results become apparent it is the 1920–40 period which is relevant to the lung cancer increase from 1940–60. It will be seen that except for the USA figures there has been little real increase in the other countries; the main spurt starts in 1945. Figures are taken with permission from: G. F. Todd, *Tobacco Research Council, Research paper No. 6*, 1963.

Curiously enough tobacco was regarded at first as having great medical value. Spanish physicians particularly recommended it for a great variety of diseases, and in 1565 Monardes, a Spanish physician, published a tome praising the weed as a kind of panacea. This very term was later used by Everardus Egidius, who published in 1587 his book *De Herba Panacea.*

We have already encountered Jean Nicot who recommended tobacco as a remedy for headaches. Other French physicians recommended it as a cure for wounds and sores as well as a remedy for incipient dropsy. William Berkeley in England advocated tobacco as a cure for a great variety of illnesses; he waxed quite lyrical and gave it as his opinion that 'It prepareth the stomach for meat; it maketh a clear voice, it maketh a sweet breath.' Many other physicians all over Europe added their praise and it remained a valued part of national pharmacopoeias until almost the beginning to the present century.

However, the advocates of tobacco didn't have it all their own way. In 1598, there appeared a tract under the title 'The Opinions of Sundry Learned Physicians' which attacked the use of tobacco in England. More famous perhaps is the tract written by James I of England in 1603, entitled 'A Counterblaste to Tobacco'. James makes fun of the notion that tobacco has any medical value and concludes that smoking is 'a custome loathesome to the Eye, hateful to the Nose, harmful to the Braine, dangerous to the Lungs, and, in the black stinking Fumes thereof, nearest resembling the horrible Stygian Smoke of the Pit that is bottomless.' This view did not find favour with all members of the Royal College of Physicians, some of whom dared to criticize their Sovereign, who in turn threatened to banish those who smoked to the country of the Red Indians.

In Italy, several Popes pronounced against the use of tobacco in Church on pain of excommunication, and in Turkey, where the smoking habit had become fashionable, the Muftis opposed it because they considered it to be contrary to the teachings of the Koran. The punishment used seems to have been rather severe; those caught smoking were dragged through the streets with the stems of their pipes pierced through the nose. Even more sadistic was Sultan Muhrad IV, who introduced the death penalty for smoking, and is reported himself to have gone out at night to catch smokers in the act. The Russians, as might have been expected, were equally cruel in the punishment they imposed on all those who violated the ban which had been proclaimed by Tsar Michael against smoking. Most of these efforts to suppress smoking took place during the seventeenth century, and other countries too attempted to introduce laws to regulate the new habit. However, very soon governments began to realize that they might profit from this new craze and many credit 'the crafty Republic of Venice' with the first imposition of financial duties, taxes and monopolies. This notion was enthusiastically followed by many other countries.

Anything that can be taxed thereby automatically becomes respectable, and most people who still attacked smoking and other uses of tobacco began to be regarded as cranks. Nevertheless, even in medical circles there was still a good deal of opposition and tobacco was made responsible for a great variety of diseases. A good example of the many evils for which smoking was blamed is contained in letters written to the Editor of the *Lancet* during 1857, partly as a consequence of some anti-smoking remarks made by Samuel Solly in an article published in that journal. Among the ailments blamed upon smoking were lunacy, cerebral haemorrhage, paralysis, delirium tremens, laryngitis, bronchitis, dyspnoea, tuberculosis, dyspepsia, gastritis, intestinal rupture, heartburn, hepatic lesions, diarrhoea, flatulence, impotence, baldness, typhoid, skin diseases and many others. The children of smokers were supposed to suffer from hypochrondriasis, hysteria and insanity. These accusations, based of course on no scientific evidence of any kind, were rebutted equally firmly by devotees of smoking, also without benefit of any scientific evidence. Many similar controversies have taken place in even quite respectable scientific journals in America, Germany, France, Italy and elsewhere. It was not in fact until the early nineteen-thirties that F. L. Hoffman in the United States and F. Lickint in Germany sounded a more serious and more scientific note by pointing to a possible association between smoking and the incidence of lung cancer.

With so many charges and countercharges flying through the air and with so many diseases being linked with smoking the question must obviously arise: how can we scientifically investigate problems of this type? How can we study these hypothetical relationships, and demonstrate clearly and unambiguously whether in fact smoking does or does not have the disastrous effects which are said to follow from it? We may note that a similar condition obtained shortly after Pasteur had discovered the existence and effects of micro-organisms. The problem arose of deciding which organisms were responsible for which diseases, and a considerable amount of confusion arose until Koch formulated his famous three postulates. These are variously quoted in textbooks on bacteriology but they may be stated fairly concisely as follows: (1) the organisms thought to be responsible for a disease must be found in all cases of the disease in question; (2) the organisms must be isolated from patients suffering from the disease and grown in pure culture; (3) when the pure culture is inoculated in susceptible animals or man it must reproduce the disease. It will be seen immediately that we are not satisfied with the simple demonstration that bacteria of a certain kind exist in people suffering from a particular disease. An organism may be present in all cases of a certain disease and yet not cause it. It is possible, for instance, that the presence of the organism may be the effect rather than the cause of the disease; some organisms have a predisposition for diseased tissue, for instance. It is also possible that the organism may simply exist as a kind of 'satellite' of another organism which might be the true cause. It is in order to differentiate between organisms which are directly responsible for a disease, and others which, although themselves present, do not cause it, that the second and third postulates were formulated. They establish that the organism is indeed the essential cause of the disease; in other words, that it has the capacity of causing the disease in question. Furthermore, the third postulate satisfies a further requirement, namely that of the proper sequence of events; to show that there is a cause-and-effect relationship between the organism and the disease we must show not only that both co-exist but that the organism preceded the disease. Bacteriologists uniformly accept the desirability of abiding by these postulates in their investigations, although it is not always possible to satisfy all three. The position is very clearly put by G. S. Wilson and A. A. Miles when they say '. . . it must be recognized that any omission in the complete chain of evidence involves a risk of error; and much confusion has been caused by uncritical attempts to support the claims advanced on behalf of numberless bacteria isolated from different parts of the body in various diseases.'[2]

Koch's three principles therefore supply us with two essential types of evidence of a link between a causal agency and a disease. The first type of evidence relates to the simultaneous presence of organism and disease and their appearance in the correct sequence, while the second relates to the specificity of effect of the organism on the development of the disease. How is all this relevant to chronic diseases such as lung cancer and coronary thrombosis where clearly infection through micro-organisms is not involved? Here we have to rely on the so-called epidemiological method of study to a far greater extent. Epidemiological investigations are differentiated from experimental ones by the fact that the epidemiological method makes use of observations of unplanned events as they occur in life, with little if any interference on the part of the investigator. In the experimental method, on the other hand, the investigator manipulates and creates a situation, usually in the laboratory, which leads to a much greater confidence in the validity of his results. Consider as an example the famous studies carried out by Snow in his work on discovering the mode of transmission of cholera. He noted that the victims during one particular outbreak tended to cluster round a particular area and he also noted that the approximate centre of this area was the Broad Street pump. The same London area was also served by another water company and households served by this company did not on the whole contact cholera. He formulated the hypothesis, therefore, that cholera was transmitted through strongly polluted water from the Broad Street pump, and he investigated this possibility very carefully in a variety of ways. For instance, he would interrogate people suffering from cholera but living at a considerable distance from the Broad Street pump, only to discover that they particularly liked the strong tasting water from this pump and had come a long way in order to obtain it. He finally removed the handle from the Broad Street pump and brought the cholera epidemic to a conclusion. This is a very famous case of an epidemiological investigation which in fact succeeded in demonstrating the causal factor and removing it.

As another example, consider the work of Goldberger on pellagra. The fact that this disease occurred frequently among sailors suffering from dietary deficiencies suggested that these might be responsible, and that pellagra might be a deficiency disease. However, this was only the first step. Epidemiological investigations can suggest a particular factor as being implicated in a particular disease but they cannot give us proof of this association. A second step is necessary, namely the demonstration by experimental means or laboratory evidence of the mode of transmission through which this particular agent exerts its effects, and thirdly the actual identification of the specific agent which causes the disease. Thus Goldberger's original epidemiological investigations were followed by experimental work in hospital wards and in prisons where experimental dietary changes could be introduced; this work constitutes the second or experimental laboratory investigation, and it provided sound proof of the dietary hypothesis. The third stage was not reached until many years later when nicotinic acid was identified as the specific agent concerned in the development of pellagra.[3].

The two cases quoted above are very well known, but they may easily give the wrong impression. In both cases the original hypothesis based on epidemiological data was in fact correct, and the reader may imagine that this is always so. The facts unfortunately are rather different. There are many first-rate epidemiological investigations implicating quite irrelevant factors. Going back to the case of pellagra, for instance, the Thompson-McFadden Commission suggested a contagion factor on the basis of their very well considered and extensive epidemiological studies; they 'recommended most heartily the installation of sanitary systems of sewage disposal as an important means of restricting the spread of pellagra.' As regards cholera, William Farr carried out a well-conceived series of epidemiological studies which led him to the conclusion that the most important factor in the transmission of this disease was the elevation above sea level, and he accordingly recommended that people should be moved to the higher inland districts and that 'armies would do better to march through the hills rather than to take the easy road over lowlands and marshes.' He also suggested that 'it would be a great advantage if soldiers in the field could sleep in raised camp beds'. We now know that Goldberger and Snow were correct and that Thompson and McFadden, and William Farr, were wrong, but at the time there was nothing to indicate that the work of the former was superior to that of the latter. In other words epidemiological investigations can give wrong conclusions as readily and as easily as correct ones, and there is nothing in the manner in which the investigation is carried out which will tell us whether the solutions are acceptable or not.

It is also interesting to note that the recommendations based upon such investigations may be followed by practical action, but that this practical action also may fail to indicate whether the original hypothesis was correct or not. Let us assume that William Farr's suggestion had been followed and that the population of London had been evacuated to the higher inland districts. Had this been done the cholera epidemic would have stopped because in fact the population would have been removed from the true cause, namely the polluted water supply. The success of the practical measures taken on the basis of a false hypothesis might then quite easily have been adduced as grounds for believing that the hypothesis was in fact correct. This, however, would have been a definite set-back because it would have made an understanding of the correct mode of transmission of cholera very much more difficult. We may say, in effect, that epidemiological investigations provide us only with circumstantial evidence, and every reader of detective stories knows the dangers involved in relying exclusively on circumstantial evidence. Epidemiological studies are only the first step and the other two steps, the experimental evidence of mode of transmission and the identification of the specific agents involved are required before we can be certain of our grounds. In saying this, of course, I have no desire to detract from the importance of this first step and the epidemiological method in general. Quite clearly in science we must have an idea before we can begin to experiment on it, but it must also be emphasized that to have an idea is not the same thing as to prove it. Compelling proof is often very difficult to achieve in these matters but we should never rest content with anything short of it.[4]'

How are all these complicated considerations relevant to the main question we are trying to answer, that is to say, the relation between smoking and diseases such as lung cancer, coronary thrombosis and so on? It will be obvious that the only way in which they have been investigated hitherto has been through the epidemiological method, ie it has been established that people who smoke more are also more likely to suffer from these various diseases; we will look at the detailed results in the next chapter. Even to establish this much is a very time-consuming, difficult and chancy business; we will note some of the objections that have been raised to the methods used in the third chapter. For the moment let us just consider the definition of the two terms involved in our equation, i.e. 'smoking' and 'disease'. We talk glibly about lung cancer, for instance, and have some idea that we know what we are talking about. In reality there are many different types of lung cancer, and the well-known Norwegian specialist, Leiv Kreyberg, has been able to show that there are two main distinct histological types.[5] Primary epithelial lung tumours of one type, which he calls Group 1 lung tumours, are made up of epidermoid carcinomas, and small cell anaplastic carcinomas; Group 2 lung tumours are made up of adenocarcinomas and bronchial or alveolar cell types. Kreyberg related the average amount smoked by his cancer patients to the estimated risk of contracting the disease of the sufferers from Group 1 lung cancer and those of Group 2 lung cancer; the results are given in Figure 2. It will be seen that there is no relationship whatsoever between smoking and Group 2 lung cancer, but a very

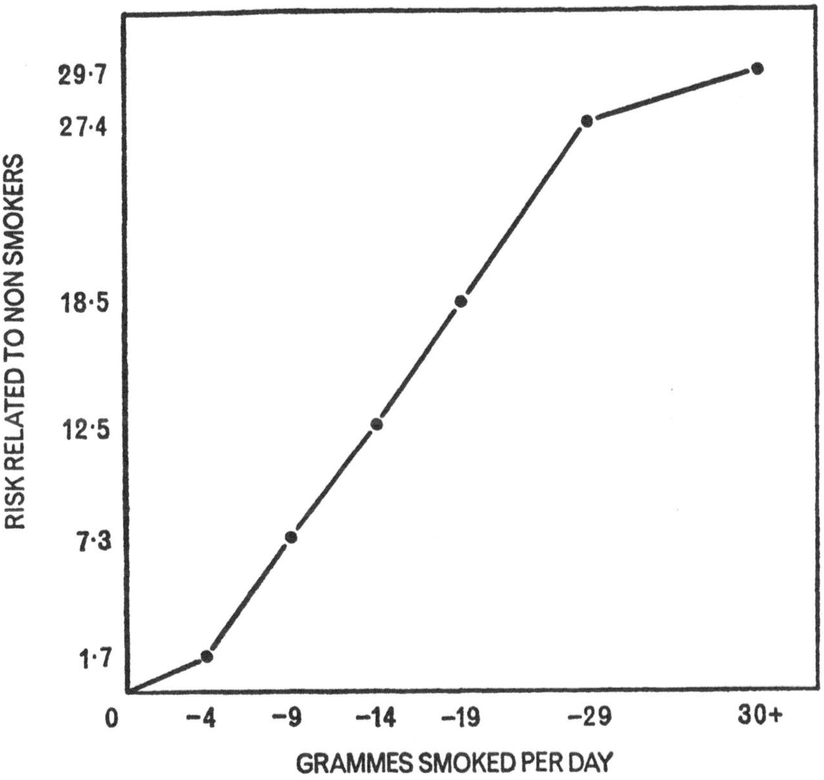

Fig. 2. Risk of contracting lung cancer of type 1 or type 2 as related to the average amount of tobacco smoked. Taken with permission from L. Kreyberg, *Brit. J. Canc.*, 1961, 15, 52.

marked straightline relationship between smoking and Group 1 lung cancer; the more tobacco is smoked per day the greater is the likelihood of developing Group 1 lung cancer. Thus lung cancer clearly is just not one undifferentiated entity; we are dealing with presumably at least two and possibly more quite different types of disease and each of these different types has different relations to smoking. Until our understanding of the disease itself is much further advanced than it is at the moment, we cannot feel very secure in our limited knowledge of this side of the equation.[6]

Let us next take smoking, and particularly cigarette smoking. Most of us will say that we know reasonably well what is meant by saying that Mr Smith smoked a cigarette, but in actual fact we know very little about the details of what is going on. As this point is crucial for much of our later discussion let me go into it in some detail. First of all we must make a distinction between what is called the *mainstream*, that is to say the smoke produced when air is sucked through the partly burning tobacco in the cigarette, and the *sidestream*, which is the smoke that arises from the tobacco when the cigarette is held in the hand or left in the ashtray. These two kinds of smoke differ very markedly in composition. Even when we consider only the mainstream there are still many variables which determine the precise chemical composition of the smoke. Some of these variables are the intensity of the suction applied, the length of the pull, the length of the interval between pulls, and the particular part of the cigarette which is being smoked, i.e. whether it is the first inch or the last inch of the cigarette. Thus what we in fact inhale depends very much on the way in which we smoke a cigarette, and it is quite impossible to generalize in any sensible way without knowing more about these different variables we have enumerated. Yet it is extremely difficult to find out precisely how cigarettes are being smoked by most people. Experiments have been conducted by simply asking people to sit in front of the experimenter and to smoke in the way they usually do; the experimenter would then take notes and calculate averages of his sample. Unfortunately, this method doesn't work at all because the unfortunate guinea pig, deprived of any other occupation but sitting there smoking, will tend to smoke much more heavily, rapidly and determinedly than he would do ordinarily. In fact, it has often been found that under those conditions there is a considerable degree of intoxication which is very rare under ordinary circumstances.

To show how little we know about these quite elementary facts the reader, if he is a cigarette smoker, may ask himself just how many pulls he takes on his cigarette on the average, and also how many pulls he thinks other people whom he knows well take. Most people imagine that they smoke at the rate of about four pulls per minute but when people are actually made to smoke at that rate they very rapidly develop severe intoxication. By observing people smoking under ordinary conditions and without any thought of being observed it has been found that the average interval between pulls was about one minute giving a rate over all of only about ten pulls from any one cigarette.

Again drawing on his experience the reader may like to ask himself just how long the pull itself might take on the average. Here again it has been found that there is a wide range of differences from a minimum of about half a second to a maximum of about four seconds. Variations of this kind make a very great deal of difference to the total quantity of smoke inhaled and also to the composition of that smoke. The same is true of the force of suction applied. Differences here from minimum to maximum were of the order of about ten times. Taking these variables together we can arrive at some rough estimate of the total volume of smoke inhaled during each pull. This seems to vary from something like 25 cc to something like 60 cc, with the average lying somewhere between 40 and 50 cc.

As we puff away the smoke is drawn through the butt of the cigarette and some of the chemicals in the smoke are filtered through this process and deposited in the butt. Consequently the last few inches of the cigarette are very much more likely to contain chemicals dangerous to health and it becomes important therefore to know just how far down the cigarette is smoked before it is thrown away. Many figures have been given of the length of cigarette stubs but even here, where one might imagine that objective measurement would be relatively easy, there are surprising differences. However, it seems to be fairly well agreed nowadays that the average length of a cigarette butt in the United States is about 1 to 2 inches and in England 0·70 inches. The figures for the Netherlands seem to be rather similar to the British ones although slightly larger. However that may be, we see that simply to say that a given person smoked a cigarette is by no means to be very informative. Even if we leave out the very important factor of inhaling we are still left with many differences between one person and another. Miss Smith may take three or four pulls of her cigarettes each of about half a second in duration and of relatively slight force, and throw away the cigarette half smoked. Mr Jones may take twenty pulls or so each of four seconds in duration and with considerable force; he may smoke his cigarette right down to the last half-inch. It is true to say in one way that both these people smoked a cigarette, but the result as far as the absorption of certain chemicals in the mainstream are concerned would be quite dissimilar. This point should be borne in mind throughout our discussion. We can ask people how many cigarettes they smoke and we may even get a fairly truthful answer. However, we cannot ask them just how they smoke these cigarettes because they themselves would be unable to give us a reasonable answer, and we cannot find out by observing them either because the very act of observation would make them change their pattern of behaviour. Under these circumstances all statistics relating to smoking must be regarded with considerable caution. We will return to this point later on.

When we do smoke cigarettes just what is it that we inhale? Smoke of course is a gas mixture containing finely divided solid and liquid particles; it is composed for the main part of liquid droplets, i.e. it is an aerosol rather than a vapour. In the tobacco smoke nicotine is of course the principal toxic alkaloid. The proportion of it which is absorbed by the organism depends very much on the way the cigarette is smoked. Far more is absorbed when deep inhaling is practised; then the proportion of nicotine absorption goes up to something like 90 per cent. Under those conditions a typical cigarette smoker using an American type cigarette will absorb something like 2·5 mg of nicotine during the smoking of one cigarette. This may be compared with the lethal dose of nicotine which is somewhere around the 50 mg level. Smokers acquire a tolerance for nicotine and the degree of toxicity experienced depends of course also on the speed with which the nicotine is being administered, i.e. the number of pulls per minute and the other factors mentioned above. Nicotine in even quite small doses is a very powerful poison, but it also has some interesting physiological effects on the nervous system which we shall discuss later on in connection with the physiological effects of smoking.

During the combustion of tobacco carbon monoxide is formed; this is a gas which has sometimes been said to be the chief industrial poison. The amount of CO produced during the smoking of one cigarette varies from some 3 cc to about 25 cc; the speed of smoking appears to be the most important variable.

There are other toxic substances in tobacco smoke but in such small concentrations that we need hardly bother with them. There are also, however, chemical irritants which are probably more important. Among these are pyradine, volatile acids and tar-like and phenolic substances. It is these which are often considered to be most particularly implicated in the production of lung cancer. It is notable that cigarette smoke is supposed to contain twice as much tar as cigar smoke – an important finding in view of the fact that it is cigarette smoking rather than cigar smoking which is usually associated with lung cancer. The amount of tar which passes into the mainstream during the smoking of one cigarette is roughly 20 mg, not all of which of course, is retained in the lungs of the smoker. However, it has been calculated that anyone who regularly smokes 20 cigarettes a day will absorb something like 100 grams of tar a year. This, it will be agreed, is quite a lot of tar!

We have now laid the groundwork for our discussion of the relationship between smoking and disease. We have briefly discussed the origin and growth of the smoking habit; we have next considered some of the objections to it on the grounds of its dangers to health and also some of the refutations. We have then turned to a consideration of the difficulties involved in proving by epidemiological investigations the causal responsibility of any particular agent for any particular disease; and we have last of all considered the problems involved in the simple definition of the act of smoking and the nature of the disease involved. With this knowledge in our hands we may now turn to the next chapter which is given over to a discussion of the many studies which have linked smoking on the one hand and lung cancer and coronary disease on the other.

Chapter 2

The Development of Suspicion

Ods me, I marvel what pleasure or felicity they have in taking their roguish tobacco. It is good for nothing but to choke a man, and fill him full of smoke and embers.

BEN JOHNSON

THE MAIN TASK of the epidemiologist is to discover variables which are always or nearly always found in conjunction with a disease in which he is interested. Quite a curious selection of variables has been found to be associated with lung cancer. Among them are sex, age, marital status, country of birth and residence, population density, social class, occupation, air pollution, smoking, consumption of alcohol, consumption of coffee, consumption of cooked shell fish and crustacea, hairiness of the second phalanges of the fingers and toes, number of teeth lost, familial factors, past history of respiratory disease, being gassed in the 1914–18 War, the number of doctors per square mile, the purchase of petrol lighters and the possession of an extraverted temperament. Of all these possible causes smoking has from the beginning been singled out. Why?

Interest in the problem began probably from a consideration of the vast increase in the number of deaths from cancer during the last sixty years. Figure 3 shows the growth of the number of cancer deaths in thousands from 1900 to 1960 in the United States. Some of this increase is simply due to a growth of the total population. Some of it is due to an increase in the age of the population. But the major part of the increase, as will be seen, is not due to any such external factors. Clearly we

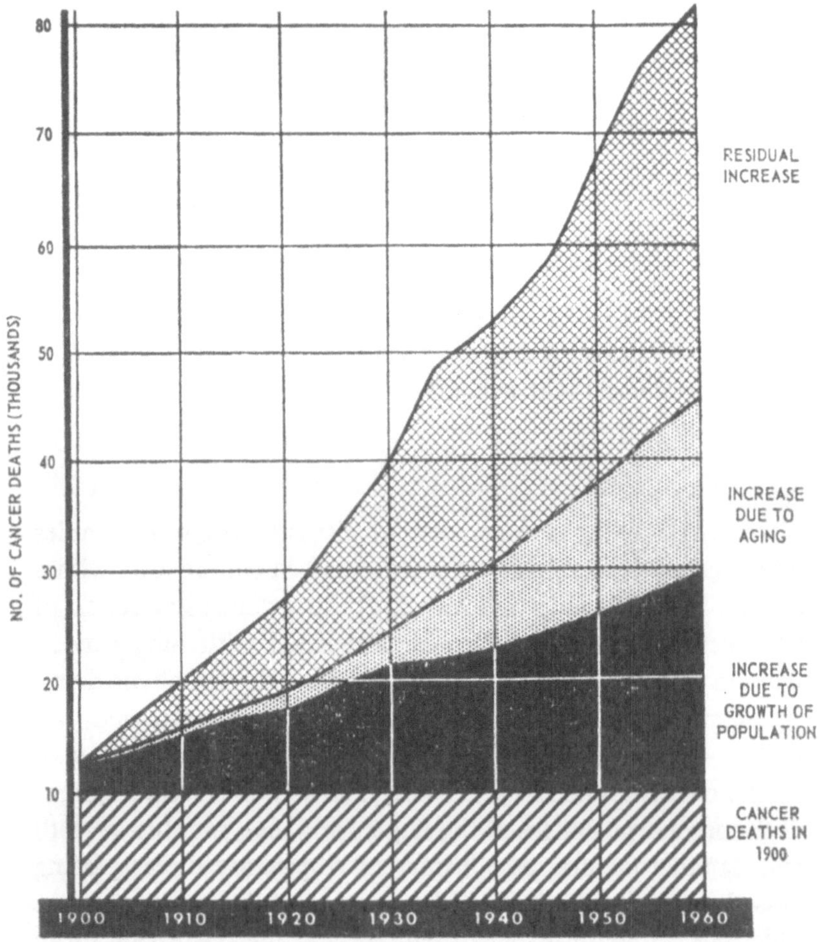

Fig. 3. Mortality rates from cancer (all types). US Death Registration Area of 1900, 1900–60. Taken with permission from 'Smoking and Health', a report of the US Department of Health, Education and Welfare.

have here a very real and terrifying problem to deal with.

However, the problem is a little more specific than that. Figure 4 shows that during the years from 1916 to 1959 the deaths of men aged 45 to 64 have been declining as far as cancer

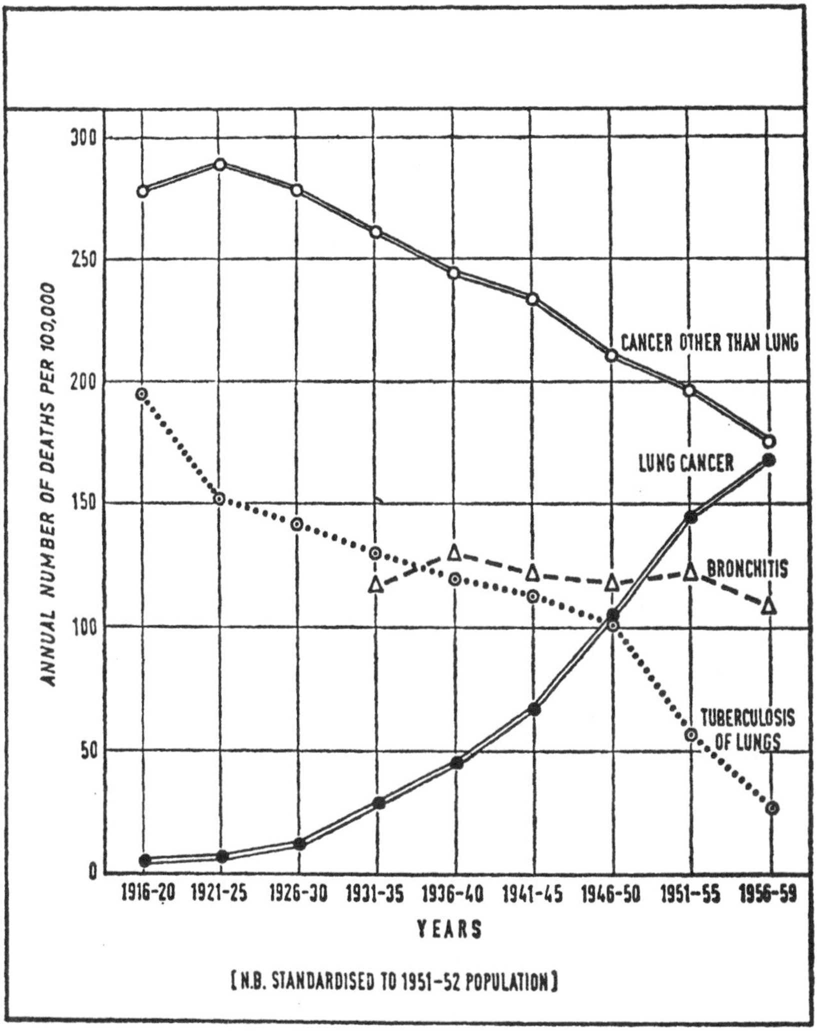

Fig. 4. Death rates from lung cancer, other forms of cancer, tuberculosis of the lungs and bronchitis, in men aged 45–64 from 1916–59. Taken with permission from 'Smoking and Health', a report of the Royal College of Physicians.

other than lung cancer is concerned just as they have been declining for tuberculosis of the lung. Bronchitis has remained pretty steady, but lung cancer has shown a phenomenal increase.

The annual number of deaths per 100,000 of the population was very near to the zero point in 1916 but rose to something like 170 in the period 1956 to 1959. Clearly something very special has been happening in the field of lung cancer and it behoves us to look for a special reason for this tremendous increase.

The growth in the consumption of tobacco particularly in the form of cigarettes appears at first sight to parallel very closely the growth in the development of lung cancer. Figure 5 shows the increase in consumption of cigarettes by both men and women, and also for men of all forms of tobacco. If we assume that the effects of smoking take a number of years to manifest themselves it would seem that the two curves, that for the increase in deaths from lung cancer and that for the increase in number of cigarettes smoked, agree very well. It is this agreement probably which sparked off the early investigations although it seems obvious that the close physical proximity of the lungs to the smoke inhaled from the cigarette must also have drawn attention to this particular variable.

Some pathologists have thrown doubt on the figures for the increase in number of deaths from lung cancer and have pointed out that the disease used to be more common than the figures suggest and that in part at least the increase may be due to the improved accuracy of diagnosis. There may be something in this objection, but it is very doubtful whether it can account for all the increase that has been observed. In particular this objection fails to account for the much faster rate of increase of lung cancer in men than in women. In the 1916–20 period there were in England and Wales 146 deaths of cancer of the lung in men and 87 in women, when we restrict ourselves to the age range of 45 to 64. From 1956 to 1959 the figures were 9,108 as compared to 1,202. This is an increase five times as great for men than for women. Clearly something else is at work besides the possibility of improved diagnosis, and clearly the situation calls for extensive inquiries of a more direct nature.

At first investigators concentrated on what are sometimes

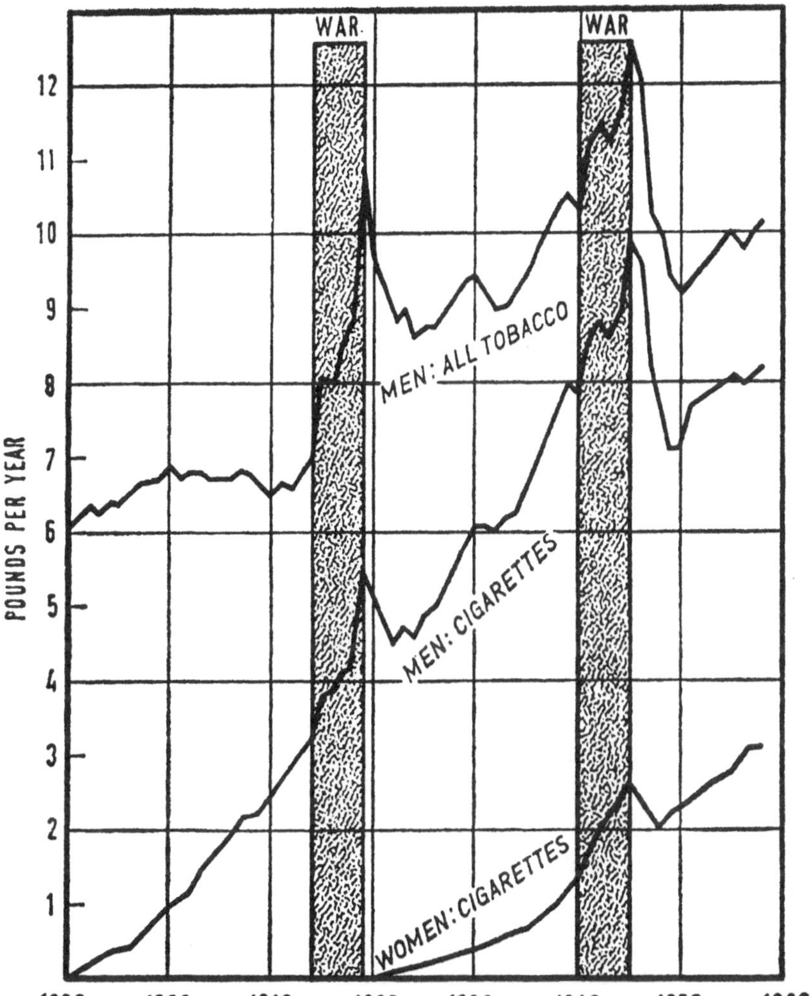

Fig. 5. Tobacco consumption in the United Kingdom from 1890–1958. This figure is taken with permission from 'Smoking and Health', a report of the Royal College of Physicians.

called 'retrospective' studies of which there are now some twenty-five in existence covering nine different countries. Essentially these studies make use of the following method. Patients with lung cancer are questioned about their smoking habits and their answers are compared with those given by individuals without lung cancer. There are many ways in which such investigations are open to criticism. Obviously we must be careful to match the lung cancer patients and the controls with respect to variables such as sex, age, social status, background, education and many other factors. This may be difficult because we cannot be sure which factors are important. Another source of inaccuracy may be that memory of one's smoking habits cannot be trusted implicitly. Another criticism is that memories of people in hospital suffering from a dread disease such as lung cancer may for various emotional reasons be falsified in one direction or the other. It has also been suggested that the interviewers might have been aware of the diagnosis and may have been influenced in their estimation of the amounts smoked by cancer patients and controls by their previously formulated hypotheses. It is unlikely that these criticisms have very much value and it is notable that a great majority of the studies carried out using this method have given results which were very similar indeed. They all agreed that among sufferers from lung cancer there is a much higher proportion of heavy smokers and a lower proportion of light smokers or of non-smokers than exists in the control groups. However, it might still be possible that the similarity of results might be due to the fact that similar errors were committed by the different investigators, and a different type of study was clearly desirable.

This other type of study has been called 'prospective'; in investigations of this type a certain population group is first defined and its smoking habits established. The members of this group are then followed up over several years and the causes of death established for each member. There are seven studies of this type, the first of which was begun in October 1951 and the latest in October 1959. The first of these was started by Drs Doll and Hill and dealt with British doctors to whom a questionnaire had been sent. All the other six are American apart from one which is Canadian; the populations for these were selected in many different ways. In all these studies questions were asked regarding the current amount and type of smoking at the time the questionnaire was answered, i.e. at the commencement of the investigation. For people who had stopped smoking previous to this point data were usually obtained on the maximum amount previously smoked per day. Care was taken to adjust the figures for differences in age distribution and other necessary statistical manipulations were carried out on the data. There would be little point in going into these details now as they are of a technical nature and it is universally agreed that the methods used are beyond criticism.[7]

The results of the 'prospective' studies agree with the 'retrospective' studies that people who die of lung cancer are precisely those who have smoked heavily for a long time. Smoking of cigars and of pipes does not seem to be associated with lung cancer to anything like the same extent, if at all. It is on these figures that the whole argument implicating smoking and lung cancer has been erected and there can be no doubt any longer that there is a statistical association between smoking and lung cancer. However, we must note at once that a statistical association or 'correlation' as it is technically known does not tell us anything about the causal relations involved. To know that A and B are correlated does not tell us whether A has caused B, B has caused A, C has caused both A and B, or whether an even more complex causal chain is involved. The point is brought out very clearly in the well-known story of a little German village where there was an almost perfect correlation between the presence of newborn babies in a house and storks on the roof. This correlation was not due to the storks being responsible for the delivery of the babies; it was due rather to a superstition obtaining in this village that storks brought good luck when a baby was expected. They were even thought to help the prospective parents to have children. Consequently any couple that wanted to have children would put up a stork nest on the roof so that the desire to have children was the causal factor in attracting the storks to that particular home.

Particularly dangerous in this connection are correlations

over time. If you plot on graph paper a large number of quite divergent variables from 1900, say, to 1960 you will find that there are very close relationships between many of them. Suppose you plot the export of pig iron from Liverpool, the number of registered prostitutes in Tokyo and the number of car tyres retreaded in Buffalo, USA; you will find that the lines are in almost perfect agreement. Nevertheless hardly anyone would suggest that there was any direct causal influence of the number of prostitutes in Tokyo on the retreading of tyres in Buffalo or the export of pig iron from Liverpool! The answer, of course, is that in the last sixty years or so there has been a population explosion leading to an increase in the production and consumption of goods. Clearly correlations will be found between all of these over this period of time, and all of these have indeed a causal relationship but it is not a direct one. The famous American psychologist, L. L. Thurstone, once said that *a correlation coefficient is a confession of ignorance*, meaning that to know only that two variables are correlated means that we are ignorant of the true causal relation between them; the knowledge of the correlation simply poses a problem, it does not give us an answer. Direct experimental evidence is required before we can accept a correlation as anything but a suggestion of a possible causal relation.

This point is so important that we may with advantage consider another example. Let us suppose that we wish to investigate the hypothesis that neurotic disorders are the product of broken homes. We might take a thousand patients diagnosed as neurotics and compare them with another thousand people who are known not to be suffering from any neurotic illness. We would investigate the home circumstances of these people and we might indeed find that the neurotics tended to come from broken homes more frequently than our non-neurotic subjects. Would this prove that broken homes are in fact responsible for later neurosis? The answer, of course, is no. There are many other possibilities that might be considered. It is possible, and indeed very likely, that neurotic disorders depend very much on inherited genetic factors, so that our present-day neurotics tend to be the children of neurotic parents. Neurotic parents in turn might be assumed to have greater difficulties in keeping their home going and are more likely therefore to (*a*) produce neurotic children and (*b*) break up their home life. On this hypothesis then the association between broken homes and neurosis in the children would not be a direct one but would be mediated by a genetic factor. There are, of course, other possibilities. It might be, for instance, that neurotic children place such a burden on the home life of their parents that a break-up is unavoidable. These various hypotheses differ, of course, in degree of *a priori* probability, but they cannot be dismissed out of hand, and we cannot come to any rational conclusion as to which is right without having much further evidence.

Is there any other evidence we have of an association between cigarette smoking and lung cancer? Figure 6 shows the relationship between cigarette consumption and the number of deaths for lung cancer in a variety of countries. The consumption figures refer to 1930, the lung cancer figures for 1950; this is done because a period of at least twenty years has to elapse before the results of the earlier smoking can be assumed to issue in deaths from lung cancer. It will be seen that there is quite a reasonable association between the two variables; as cigarette consumption increases so does the number of deaths from lung cancer. Roughly speaking the figures suggest that 50 per cent of the differences in lung cancer deaths from one country to another are due to the differences in cigarette consumption. Some countries lie suspiciously far away from the main regression line which has been drawn through the cluster of points. The United States of America, for instance, has too few deaths for its rate of cigarette consumption, and Great Britain has too many. It may be possible that this is due to the fact that in Great Britain a greater part of the cigarette is consumed than in the United States, where butts tend to be much longer, as we have seen. Another possibility is the higher proportion of young people in the United States population.

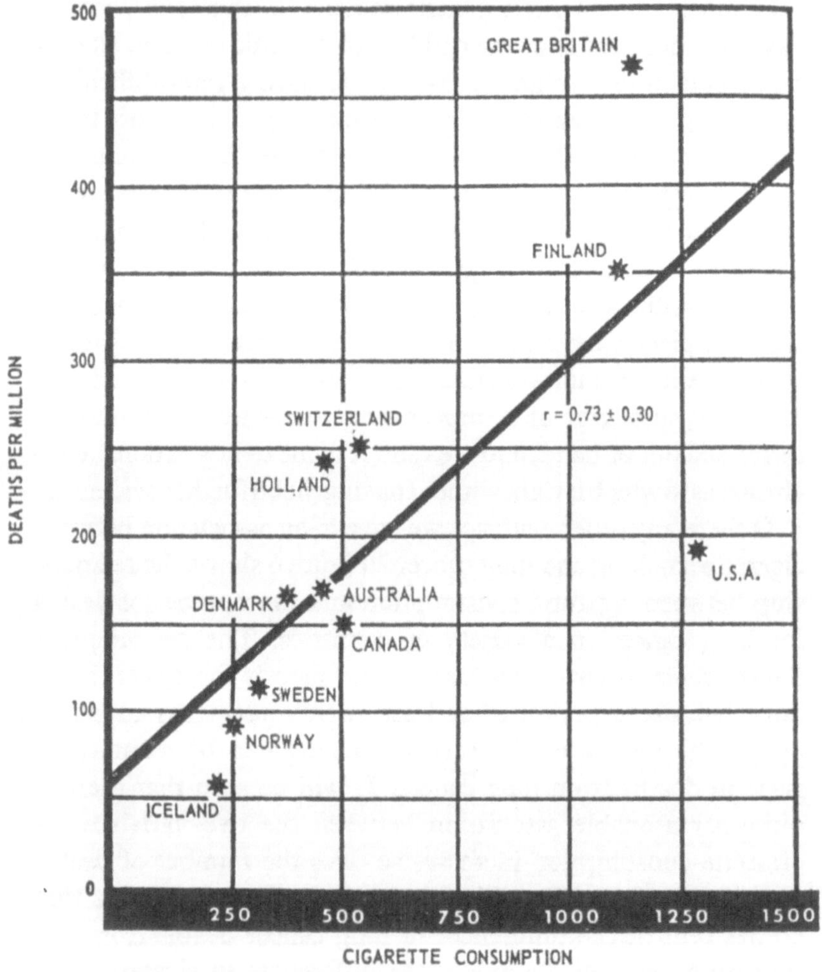

Fig. 6. Crude male death rate for lung cancer in 1950 and per capita consumption of cigarettes in 1930 in various countries. This figure is taken with permission from 'Smoking and Health', a report of the US Dept. of Health, Education and Welfare.

The figures are certainly interesting and in line with those presented before, but they still represent a correlation and nothing more; no direct causal argument can be based on these figures. [8]

While lung cancer has had most of the limelight as far as smoking is concerned it is by no means the only disease that is implicated in connection with smoking. Doll and Hill in their investigation of British doctors found a considerable increase in coronary death rates with increasing tobacco consumption but they failed to demonstrate any marked differences between non-smokers, light and heavy smokers among the older men. American findings, too, suggest that the main correlation between smoking and coronary disease occurs during early middle age. Figure 7 is taken from the American prospective study by Hammond and Horn and shows the death rate from coronary heart disease in American men aged 50 to 70 when smokers are compared with ex-smokers and non-smokers. It will be seen that ex-smokers seem to have a rather better expectancy of life than do people who have continued to smoke and this finding is very much in line with what has been found in relation to lung cancer too. There ex-smokers tend to resemble non-smokers more than they do heavy smokers as far as risk of death is concerned, although, of course, length of time during which the habit has been given up is an important variable.

Table 1 shows the total number of expected and observed deaths and mortality ratios for smokers of cigarettes. The figures were taken from the seven prospective studies referred to previously, and the mortality ratios indicate the increased likelihood of dying from a particular disease for cigarette smokers. It will be seen that there are increased probabilities of death for quite a variety of different disorders ranging from an increase of about 1,100 per cent for cancer of the lung to 50 per cent for cancer of the kidney. Also given in this table are the actual differences between the number of smokers dying of a disease and the number of people expected to die of the disease at that particular age. It will be seen that while cancer of the lung is top of the table as far as the mortality ratios are concerned, it is far outstripped by coronary artery disease as far as the actual differences between expected and observed number of deaths are concerned. This, of course, is due to the fact that far more

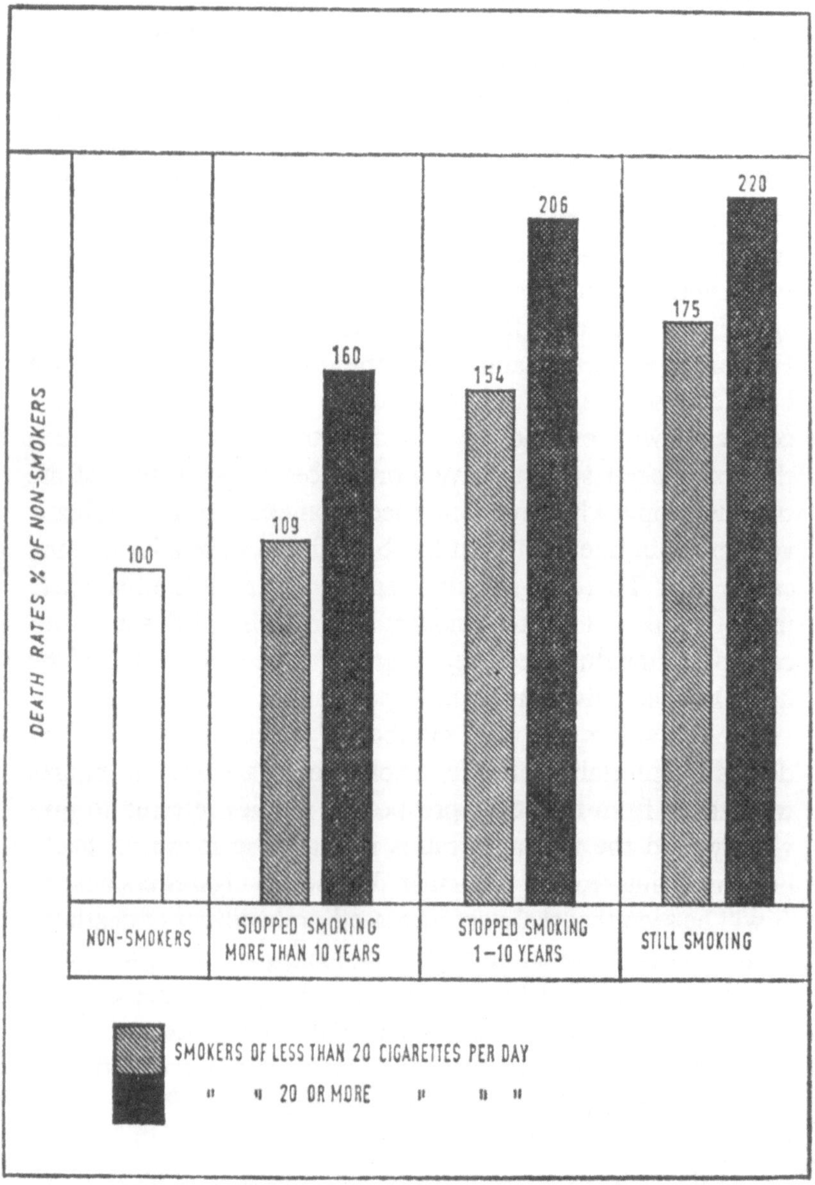

Fig. 7. The relationship of death rates from coronary heart disease to smoking habits. This figure is taken by permission from 'Smoking and Health', a report of the Royal College of Physicians.

TABLE I

	Expected	*Observed*	*D*	*Mortality Ratio*
Cancer of the lung	170	1,833	1,657	10·8
Bronchitis and emphysema	90	546	456	6·1
Cancer of the larynx	14	75	61	5·4
Cancer of oral cavity	37	152	115	4·1
Cancer of oesophagus	34	113	79	3·4
Stomach and duodenal ulcers	105	294	189	2·8
Other circulatory diseases	254	649	395	2·6
Cirrhosis of liver	169	379	210	2·2
Cancer of bladder	112	216	104	1·9
Coronary artery disease	6,431	11,177	4,746	1·7
Other heart diseases	526	868	342	1·7
Hypertensive heart disease	409	631	222	1·5
General arteriosclerosis	211	310	99	1·5
Cancer of kidney	79	120	41	1·5
All other cancer	1,061	1,524	463	1·4
Cancer of stomach	285	413	128	1·4
Influenza, pneumonia	303	415	112	1·4
All other causes	1,509	1,946	437	1·3
Cerebral vascular lesions	1,462	1,844	382	1·3
Cancer of prostate	253	318	65	1·3
Accidents, suicides, violence	1,063	1,310	247	1·2
Nephritis	156	173	17	1·1
Rheumatic heart disease	291	309	18	1·1
Cancer of rectum	208	213	5	1·0

Adapted from figures published in the American Report. The heading 'Observed' refers to actual deaths in the population under study; 'Expected' refers to deaths among non-smokers. Column 'D' gives the absolute difference between the two first columns; thus 4,746 more persons died of coronary artery disease than would have been expected to do so if they had none of them smoked. The column headed 'Mortality Ratio' gives the ratio Observed/Expected; in the case of lung cancer this is 10·8, indicating that almost eleven times as many people died of this disease than would have been expected to do so if none had smoked.

people die of coronary disease than of cancer of the lung, and this difference more than makes up for the greater increase in probability of dying associated with smoking.[9]

Experts are divided as to whether a causal role should be claimed for smoking in the causation of coronary heart disease. There are certain important similarities as far as this disease and lung cancer are concerned, but there are also certain differences. Lung cancer, for instance, is rare in non-smokers. The disease is associated with cigarette smoking at all ages and no characteristic other than smoking has been demonstrated to increase liability to it. Coronary heart disease on the other hand frequently affects non-smokers. The association with smoking seems to be clear only in middle age, and various other factors, such as sedentary occupation, indulgence in fatty foods and mental strain have been suggested to increase liability to coronary thrombosis. More recently sugar too has been implicated. Nevertheless, these factors themselves are in part related to heavy smoking, and it has recently been shown that there is a significant relationship between coronary heart disease and inhaling during smoking. Clearly the question of a causal implication is still open.

There would be little point in quoting at great length the many other diseases where it has been shown that smoking is correlated with the development of the disorder. Many of these diseases are relatively rare and most readers would not be likely to have any significant knowledge of them. Furthermore full details are given in the British report [10] and the American report on the association between smoking and disease. However, the figures for all these different diseases may be taken together and plotted, as has been done in Figure 8. This figure, which has been derived from one of the prospective studies mentioned before, shows the death rates per 10,000 men years for smokers and non-smokers at various ages. It will be noted that the death rates are given in logarithmic form in order to get all the data on to one sheet. It will also be noticed that the two lines are not parallel but tend to converge; this indicates that the mortality ratio is declining with increased age. To put this finding in a rather different way we might say that if you have survived to the age of 70 or above your chances of dying are not increased as much by your previous smoking history as they might have been if you were only 40 or 50. Whichever way we look at this figure, however, the contrast is fairly startling. At the age of 47·5 non-smokers have only half the death rate of smokers and while this difference declines as age increases, it still remains quite noticeable even at the highest ages plotted. It would seem that either smoking has a lot to answer for, or else that people who are generally unhealthy tend to indulge in smoking more than do healthy ones. We notice again that all that has been established is a statistical association or correlation; we cannot immediately decide from looking at these figures what causal relation there may be between smoking and death from disease.

It will be noted that the differences between smokers and non-smokers can be defined more rigorously to exclude light smokers. Mortality ratios for current smokers of cigarettes go up as the amount smoked increases. In the study of British doctors, for instance, which was carried out by Doll and Hill, the ratio was 1·06 when less than 10 cigarettes were smoked per day. It rose to 1·31 when between 10 and 20 were smoked, to 1·62 when between 20 and 34 were smoked, and to 2·50 when more than 35 were smoked. Similar figures are given for the various American studies. Ratios for cigar smokers are throughout much lower. They are not raised at all above 1 when less than 5 are smoked; when more than 5 are smoked the mortality ratio goes up to only about 1·2. For pipes again the over-all ratio remains pretty well identical with that of non-smokers, almost regardless of how many pipes are smoked per day.

This is a very brief summary of the evidence. It has been considered very carefully by two eminent medical committees. The first was set up by the Royal College of Physicians and it reported in 1962 in a publication entitled *Smoking and Health*. The committee concluded that 'Cigarette smoking is the cause of lung cancer and bronchitis and probably contributes to the

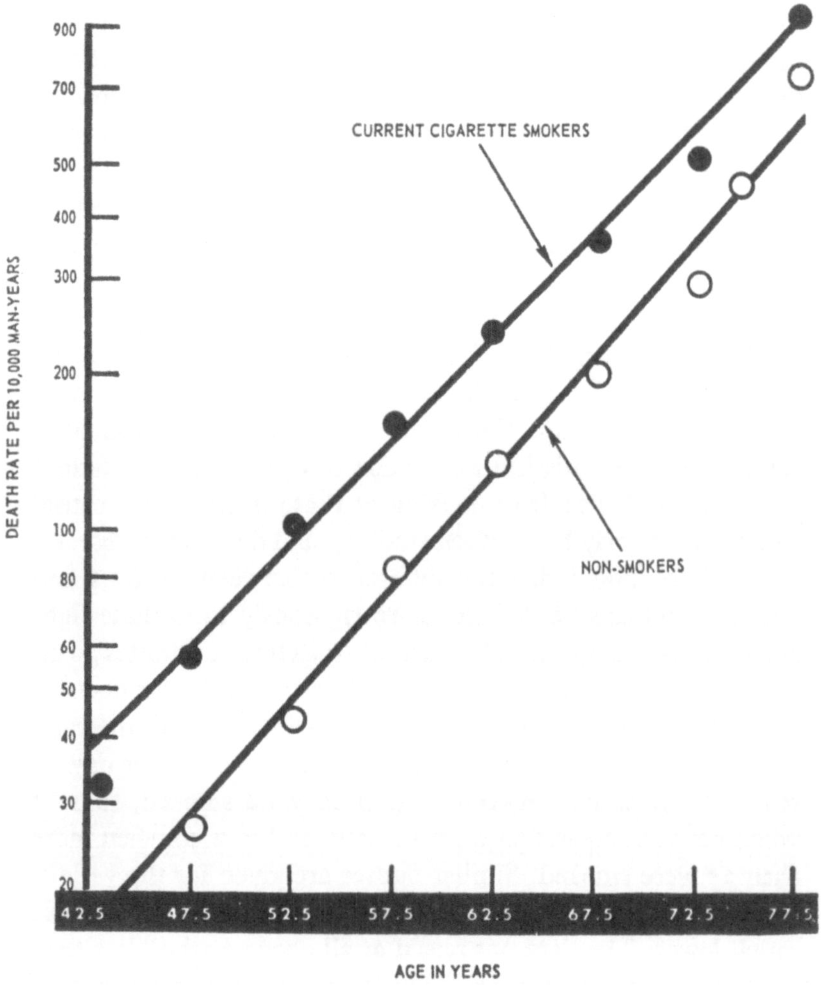

Fig. 8. Death rate (logarithmic scale) plotted against age. Taken from a prospective study of mortality in US veterans, and quoted by permission from 'Smoking and Health', a report of the US Dept. of Health, Education and Welfare.

development of coronary heart disease and various other less common diseases. It delays healing of gastric and duodenal ulcers. . . . The number of deaths caused by diseases associated with smoking is large . . . it is necessary for the health of the people in Britain that any measures that are practicable and likely to produce beneficial changes in smoking habits should be taken promptly.'

A similar report, also entitled *Smoking and Health*, was made by the Advisory Committee of the Surgeon General of the Public Health Service in the United States. The conclusions of this committee were as follows: 'Cigarette smoking is causally related to lung cancer in men; the magnitude of the effect of cigarette smoking far outweighs all other factors. The data for women, though less extensive, point in the same direction. The risk of developing lung cancer increases with duration of smoking and the number of cigarettes smoked per day; it is diminished by discontinuing smoking.' The committee then go on to state that 'the causal relationship of smoking pipes to the development of cancer of the lip appears to be established. . . . Cigarette smoking is a significant factor in the causation of laryngeal cancer in the male. . . . Cigarette smoking is the most important of the causes of chronic bronchitis in the United States, and increases the risk of dying from chronic bronchitis. . . . Male cigarette smokers have a higher death rate from coronary artery disease than non-smoking males but it is not clear that the association has causal significance.'

Here then we have a very thorough-going indictment of smoking, particularly cigarette smoking, and it is notable that both committees specially set-up for the purpose of evaluating the evidence have come to very similar, if not identical, conclusions. Yet, many individual experts have criticized the evidence on various grounds and have suggested that the causal implications of smoking have not been demonstrated as conclusively as these quotations would seem to suggest. In our next chapter we will therefore deal with some of the criticisms that have been made and try to assess their validity. We will then go on to discuss alternative hypotheses to explain the data quoted in this chapter.

Chapter 3

The Critics Hit Back

Said one – 'Folks of a surly Tapster tell,
And daub his Visage with the Smoke of Hell;
They talk of some strict Testing of us – Pish!
He's a Good Fellow, and 'twill all be well.'

EDWARD FITZGERALD

THE WORK OF Doll and Hill in England, of Horn and Hammond in America, and of all the other investigators who have taken up the trail of the disease-producing effects of cigarette smoking, has, of course, not gone unchallenged. I shall not in this chapter deal with all the arguments that have been advanced in an attempt to rebut their conclusions. Many of the criticisms are themselves unsound, and it would be a waste of time to discuss them in detail. Others, while reasonable at the time when they were made, have since been answered by the original authors, either in further analyses of their data, or by new studies. In going through the writings of Doll and Hill, and of Horn and Hammond again for the purpose of this book I was struck, as I had been when I had read them originally, by the great care which had been taken in the carrying out of these investigations, by the way in which the authors took note of published criticism and tried to answer it by adducing further factual information, and by their wholly admirable refusal to be side-tracked from strictly scientific argument. I believe that the case which they make out can be criticized but that is merely to say that scientific investigators, even the most eminent, are only human; whatever the truth of the criticisms here presented the work of these investigators will always remain as a fine example of scientific detective work.

The first point to be considered is one frequently made by Joseph Berkson, a well-known statistician associated with the Mayo Clinic in America. He put the point in the following way: 'Statistical studies even if they are free of obvious difficulties such as are manifest in the present studies are not conclusive in questions like the present one. They must be confirmed by experimental studies and other different types of investigation and this has not happened in the present case. The theory, as originally set forth, was that cigarette smoke contains carcinogenic chemicals like benzpyrene and arsenic which, in contact with the surface tissues of the lung, initiate the development of what is called squamous cell or epidermoid cancer. This type is cancer of the superficial layers of the lung tubes and it seemed plausible that smoking could have such an effect. I don't think pathologists would have considered seriously the suggestion that smoking can cause the more deep-seated adeno type of lung cancer. In support of this theory statistics have been published showing that the observed increased incidence of lung cancer was confined pretty much to the squamous cell or epidermoid type. Apparently with the expectation of corroborating this recently at the Los Angeles County Hospital a study of necropsy specimens dating back to 1927 was made. It was found that the relative proportion of epidermoid cancers is not increasing but decreasing, while the proportion of adeno type is increasing. Since the incidence of observed lung cancer in the population surveyed had increased this falsifies the generalization that whenever the observed incidence of lung cancer has increased the increase has been that of the epidermoid type.' To the question whether the theory that lung cancer is caused by carcinogens in the cigarette smoke was not valid Berkson replied: 'The suspected carcinogens like benzpyrene and arsenic were found to be in minute concentration in cigarette smoke as to be incapable of producing the cancers. Even strong contenders of the smoking/lung cancer theory no longer believe cancer is produced by carcinogens contained in tobacco smoke . . . the whole fabric of the original theory has broken down and virtually been abandoned.'

Berkson goes on to say that attempts to produce lung cancer in rats and other animals by blowing cigarette smoke at them for very long periods of time have not in fact succeeded. As he puts it: 'So far as clinical evidence is concerned I should not fail to mention here that it had been early noted by others that the notion of smoking as the cause of cancer was incongruous with clinical experience.' He specifically quotes Dr R. D. Passey who had been trying for many years without success to produce cancer of the lung in animals with smoke. After about 5 years of experiment a final definitive report was issued by Passey saying 'Our failure during the past 5 years to induce lung tumours in mice, rats and hamsters by exposure to strong concentrations of cigarette smoke is a striking negative result. In these experiments the only lung cancer encountered had been a solitary tumour in a control rat.[11]

There is then, according to Berkson, no experimental, physiological, biochemical evidence for the carcinogenic effects of cigarette smoking, but only statistical evidence. Rather mischievously he quotes a rather interesting observation from a book by Albert Schweitzer. 'On my arrival in Gabon, in 1913, I was astonished to encounter no cases of cancer. I saw none among the natives 200 miles from the coast.

'I cannot of course say positively that there was no cancer at all, but like other frontier doctors, I can only say that if any cases existed they must have been quite rare. This absence of cancer seemed to me due to the difference in nutrition of the natives as compared to the Europeans. The most significant being that the natives 200 miles from the coast consumed no salt.

'In the course of the years, we have seen cases of cancer in growing numbers in our region.

'My observations incline me to attribute this to the fact that the natives were living more and more to the manner of the whites, seasoning their meat with salt and consuming canned vegetables and meat and tinned milk, as they had not formerly done.' Berkson's comment is: 'When the cause of a disease is not known, frequently it gets attributed to practices that are not approved, like the use of alcohol perhaps, or like smoking. . . . Here we see the attribution of a causal relation between two events occurring together in time, both considered evil; cancer and canned or condimented food.' Berkson ends his survey of the writings of many advocates of the theory that smoking causes cancer by saying 'We find then in this, I hope not unfair, summary of some biologic considerations that, in advocating the theory that smoking causes cancer of the lung, pathologists do not present pathology based on their study of individual cases but statistics, the clinicians present not clinical experience with individual patients setting forth the particulars in each case that support the theory, but the same statistics . . . virtually the sole support for the theory is from statistics.'

The burden of this first criticism then is a point we have tried to make before. What has been established is a relationship but only a statistical one; whether there is a causal one, and just how such a causal relationship might work is completely undetermined. We might with advantage quote here the famous physiologist Claude Bernard: 'I do not reject the use of statistics, but I condemn not trying to go beyond them. . . .' Statistics are an interesting, important and suggestive first step in the search for an explanation of lung cancer, but they cannot in the nature of the case be more than suggestive. We need a biological link and this can only be provided by proper experimentation.

The second criticism I want to mention is also one made by Berkson. We have already drawn attention to the fact that the relationship between smoking and lung cancer is not specific but that a great number of other diseases also apparently are related to cigarette smoking. He summarizes some of the data we have already presented in Figure 9, which is quoted from one of his publications. In connection with this diagram he has the following to say: 'In the chart is presented the age adjusted death rate for each of these disease groups classified according to the amount of smoking of cigarettes. Surely it is true that there is a graded increase of the death rate from cancer of the lung with increase of amount of smoking but equally surely there is an

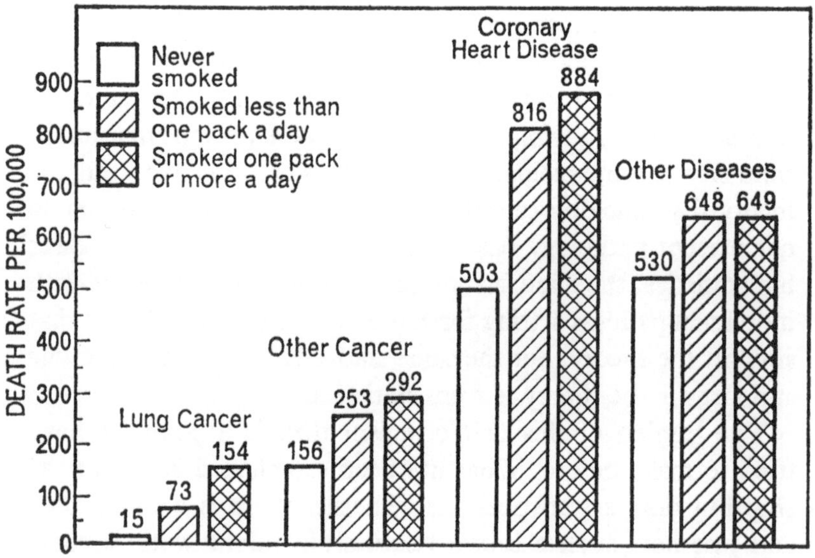

Fig. 9. Age-adjusted death rates for various disease groups in relation to amount of smoking. Taken with permission from J. Berkson, *Proc. of the Staff Meetings of the Mayo Clinic*, 1960, **35**, 374.

increase of death rate, with an increased amount of smoking, in each of the other three categories into which all causes of death have been segregated. We are presented with findings that bear no particular relation to the specific increase in death rate from cancer of the lung observed in the vital statistics records, nor to benzpyrene or arsenic or other substances in tobacco smoke acting as contact carcinogens. Something very different is on view here than was originally envisaged to explain the observed rise of death rate from cancer of the lung, but that there is a statistical association between smoking and all causes of death generally of which cancer of the lung is only a small part. We have here a great deal more than was bargained for and most of it without relation to what it was intended to explain, the observed rise in death rate from cancer of the lung. If we take the higher death rate from cancer of the lung among the smokers as evidence that smoking causes such cancer then we must also accept that smoking causes cancer of the stomach, of the bladder, of the prostate, for all of which the death rates are higher among the smokers. It is as though in investigating a drug that previously had been indicated to relieve the common cold the drug was found not only to ameliorate corryza but also to cure pneumonia, cancer and many other diseases. We have 'proved too much' and the scientists would be inclined to say 'there must be something wrong with this method of investigation.'[12]

Here Berkson is arguing, in effect, that the original hypothesis that certain carcinogens in the smoke brought into contact with the lungs produced lung cancer is an intelligible and plausible hypothesis. If smoking were shown to be related to lung cancer in this entirely specific manner then one might feel inclined to support the hypothesis. But instead, what we find is that lung cancer is only one of many disorders which are associated with cigarette smoking, and in none of the other disorders is there any question of carcinogenic agents in the smoke coming in contact with the afflicted parts. Consequently, the theory ceases to be specific and becomes so general as to be almost meaningless. Smoking by losing its specific affinity with lung cancer ceases to be an intelligible cause of lung cancer either.

There are several more or less plausible answers to this argument. One is that the causal relations between cigarette smoking and the different diseases may be quite different. Thus it is possible that carcinogenic agents in the smoke produce lung cancer, and that other elements produce debilitating effects on the smoker which make him less able to resist the ravages of other diseases. However, such alternative hypotheses would have to be spelt out in more detail than they have been hitherto in order to make this argument attractive. Another answer to Berkson, curiously enough, may be derived from quite a different line of criticism of the original studies of Doll and Hill and of Horn and Hammond, namely criticisms related to their selection of subjects. It may be argued that this selection was carried out in such a way as artificially to inflate the mortality ratios and thus make it appear that smoking is responsible for a much larger number of diseases than is actually justified by the figures. By thus stressing a rather different type of criticism we may be able to overcome some at least of the difficulties which are raised by Berkson in this argument. In order to appraise the validity of this suggestion, however, we must now turn to the third criticism which is concerned with methods of selection.

Let us have a good look at the populations which were studied in the seven prospective investigations, and which constitute the hard core of the case for the association between lung cancer and smoking. None of these studies was designed to be representative of the British or American population, and none of them is in fact even remotely representative in this sense. This is a very important qualification. We normally study a sample of people in order to be able to gain knowledge about the total population of which they are a sample, but in the case of the prospective smoking study, as the American report recognizes very well, 'any answer to the question "to what general populations of men can the results be applied?", must involve an element of unverifiable judgement.' Such 'unverifiable judgements' must, of course, cast a good deal of doubt on the statistical results which are reported. These doubts are likely to be confirmed by the finding that the death rates for non-smokers in these studies are markedly below those of US white males and that even the smokers of one pack of cigarettes or more daily have death rates that average slightly below the US white males figure. In part this may be explained by the fact that hospitalized and other seriously ill persons were not recruited in these studies, but the size of the differences is still rather surprising. An additional possibility is that there was a selection in these studies towards men of higher economic levels, whose death rates tend to be lower. Another reason given by the American report as a possibility is a failure to trace all deaths. 'In mass studies it is almost impossible to devise an infallible provision for recording every death. The study directors were, however, experienced in handling this problem and it seems unlikely that more than, say, 5 per cent of the deaths would be missed.' Five per cent may, of course, not seem a large number, but errors of this kind can be cumulative.

J. Berkson has brought out the unrepresentative nature of the samples studied in a particularly impressive fashion. In a private communication he wrote: 'If we take the observations upon the smokers and non-smokers in the "prospective studies" to represent an experiment, and this is the way they have been presented, and consider that the higher death rate among the smokers reflects excess deaths caused by smoking, then an analysis of Hammond's last paper (not yet published) shows that about every third death in the adult population in the United States is due to smoking, only about 12 per cent of these being due to lung cancer. About 50 per cent of the deaths from cancer of the pancreas, 20 per cent of deaths from cancer of the stomach, 36 per cent of deaths from leukemia, 31 per cent of deaths from heart and circulatory diseases, etc., are due to smoking on this interpretation. Even 12 per cent of deaths from accidents and violence are due to smoking according to these results. Interestingly enough, although this is the sort of result one gets if one compares the death rate of the smokers with that of the non-smokers, if one compares them with the general population, the death rates are smaller not larger – for deaths from all causes, from lung cancer and from heart disease. A similar result is obtained if one considers the comparison of deaths from all causes presented in the extraordinary Figure 1, p. 88 of the US Surgeon General's Report on Smoking and Health, representing the results of the US Veterans Study (Figure 8 in this book). Since the average 'mortality ratio' for the cigarette smokers is about 1·7, the proportion of deaths among them due to smoking is $1-1/1{\cdot}7=41$ per cent. Yet the death rates of these same smokers are much lower than that of the general population! (Table 15, p. 95 of the *American Report.*) The results of the English studies are similar though not so extreme. There, from a similar analysis, one would conclude that about one in five deaths among cigarette smokers in the adult population is caused by their smoking. Nevertheless, the death rate among these smokers is smaller than that of the comparable general population for all causes and for lung cancer.'

Even if the original sample as intended by the experimenters had been acceptable, it must be noted that these people were approached by mail and that only a relatively small proportion did in fact agree to take part in the investigation. In the British study 68 per cent agreed to take part and the figure for the American studies is rather similar. Thus we find that the respondents are very highly selected and little is known about the basis of this selection. In the British sample Doll has found that the death rate of non-respondents was higher than that of respondents and that there were more smokers among the non-respondents than among the respondents. It is possible by making certain rather arbitrary but not unreasonable assumptions to discover what effect these biases may have on mortality ratios. The conclusion appears to be that response bias in the mortality ratio might be as high as 0·3, for mortality ratios lying between 1 and 2. A mortality ratio of 5·0 might overestimate by 1·0, and one of 10·0 might overestimate by 3·0. Thus a possible result of the various sources of error in selection might be to produce a spurious raising of the mortality ratios and we might perhaps be justified therefore in disregarding those below 1·5, in Table 1. Doing this, of course, rather lowers the importance of Berkson's argument regarding the lack of specificity of lung cancer and smoking relationships by wiping out a large number of diseases which would otherwise have been found to be related to smoking. Nevertheless, some diseases still survive and lend some force to Berkson's argument.

Altogether it seems surprising that so little criticism has been directed at the refusal rate of over 30 per cent which obtains in all these prospective studies. In work on social attitudes done by academic psychologists or by organizations such as the Gallup Poll, or in market research inquiries carried out by commercial agencies, a refusal rate of even 10 per cent would cause raised eyebrows and would probably call forth serious criticism of the conclusions. In our own work we have regarded a refusal rate of 5 per cent as being the limit of what was regarded as permissible and have generally relied on data from samples where the refusal rate was more like 2 per cent.[13] Admittedly, the task of the investigators in the prospective studies of smokers and non-smokers was exceptionally difficult, but even so, such a high refusal rate cannot be condoned if serious consideration is to be given to the numerical accuracy and meaningfulness of the results. As Sir Ronald Fisher, who has been critical of the analysis of the English data on smoking and lung cancer, remarked in his book *Smoking: the Cancer Controversy* in 1959: 'The question seems to be a serious one; when is serious investigation going to begin?'

In connection with the problem of selection it is interesting to consider the relationship to death rate of a variety of variables which have been examined. Thus there is a relationship between dying and having long-lived parents and grandparents. The death rates of non-smokers with long-lived antecedents was 14·8, that of non-smokers with short-lived antecedents 21·1. Comparative figures for cigarette smokers were 27·1 and 44·8. Having or not having had a previous serious disease provided even more marked differences; the death rates were 11·5 and 42·5 for non-smokers, 22·3 and 65·0 for cigarette smokers. Single people had a higher death rate than married, 26·0 as compared to 18·9 for non-smokers, and 50·1 as compared to 33·0 for smokers. Educational level was clearly related to death rate, the figures for non-smokers ranging from 22·7 for those with the least amount of education to 15·8 for college graduates; for cigarette smokers the corresponding figures were 35·2 and

29·4. The amount of exercise too was important; dividing the population into four groups (taking no, slight, moderate or heavy exercise) the death rates for non-smokers were found to be 23·8, 14·7, 11·0 and 9·5; for cigarette smokers they were 34·1, 25·5, 20·8 and 19·7. Interesting as these figures are they do not throw much light on the controversy itself.

The last criticism to mention before we turn to what in our opinion is really the most crucial of all is one to which relatively little attention has been paid. In associating smoking and disease it is clearly essential that a very accurate assessment should be made of the amount of smoking that has taken place in the life history of every single subject. Yet, as the American report emphasizes, 'Measurement of the type and amount of smoking, being based on a single mail questionnaire, was admittedly crude.' It is quite difficult for most people to know just how much they are in fact smoking and estimates are not likely to be very reliable. More important probably is the fact that the number of cigarettes smoked is only one and may not be the most important part of the evidence that is to be considered. We have already mentioned the importance of how many pulls are taken on the cigarette, how much of it is smoked, and how strong the pull is on the average; these variables are not usually known to the smoker himself and are not inquired about in the usual type of questionnaire. We thus have only unreliable and relatively uninformative material to go on as far as the smoking side of the equation is concerned. In so far as the errors involved in ascertaining the number of cigarettes smoked are random, little mischief is probably done because such errors will tend to attenuate rather than exaggerate any association that may be present. But there may also be systematic errors in reporting the amount smoked. As the American report says: 'Heavy smokers may tend to underestimate the amount smoked. If this happens the reported increase in mortality ratio per additional cigarette smoked will be an overestimate of the true increase, although the upward trend of mortality ratio with increasing amount smoked will remain.' The authors of the report finally come to a rather comforting conclusion. They say: 'On balance, we are inclined to agree with the opinion expressed by the authors of several of the studies to the effect that the general result of errors reporting smoking history is to depress the mortality ratios of smokers relative to non-smokers, so that reported ratios will tend to be underestimates so far as this source of error is concerned.' This may be true, but no convincing evidence has been offered on this point and it is difficult to see how such evidence could be produced. In its absence one might just as easily adopt the opposite point of view and consider that the reported mortality ratios are in fact over-estimates. It is difficult to know just how important this point may be but it adds to the considerable uncertainty which exists about the figures as reported. Each of the sources of uncertainty which we have discussed so far may by itself be relatively unimportant. In conjunction, however, and particularly if all the errors should go in the same direction they may add up to a very considerable total. The difficulty is not so much that the figures as published are subject to error; all scientific measurement is subject to error and therefore these figures would not be expected to be perfect. However, what characterizes scientific measurement is that we have some notion of the probable size of the error, that is to say we can tell up to a point within which limit the true measure will lie. What is so disconcerting with these figures is that we have no notion at all, even approximately, of the size of the various errors or even their direction. Under these circumstances the figures as published assume a spurious degree of accuracy which is very misleading. Admittedly there are very great difficulties indeed in finding out the true facts, but it is necessary for the reader to realize that the true facts are not known and that all we have are very rough and ready approximations which are subject to varying, possibly large, degrees of error which themselves cannot be estimated in the majority of instances. Just what the true figures might be if all these sources of error were removed we cannot at present even guess.

More fundamental, and probably more important, than any of the criticisms so far considered is one which has been made by several people but most persistently and most strongly perhaps by J. Yerushalmy, a biostatistician associated with the University of California.[14] Yerushalmy begins by saying that 'A strong association has been demonstrated between cigarette smoking and cancer of the lung.' He then considers some of the criticism of biased sampling which have been made of these studies, and continues: 'However, if the association were due entirely to these sampling biases they would not have persisted for many years after the initiation of the investigation. The fact that cigarette smokers continued to have higher rates in the second and third year of observation would indicate that the association between cigarette smoking and cancer of the lung is not a resultant of these sampling peculiarities alone. Consequently, the association itself is accepted as definitely established. The question turns to the interpretation of this association in terms of causation.'

Yerushalmy next turns to the main point of his criticism which is that the samples were not chosen randomly or independently, but are *self-selected*. 'The main difficulty in evaluating such association stems from the fact that the individuals observed have made for themselves the crucial decision whether they are smokers, non-smokers or past-smokers. Consequently, the groups lack the comparability necessary for definitive experimentation.' This criticism can best be understood by first of all looking at a hypothetical experiment which would not be subject to this criticism. In such an ideal investigation we would have, say, 7,000 volunteers of whom we randomly allocate 1,000 to a non-smoking group, another 1,000 to a group smoking no more than 10 cigarettes a day, another 1,000 to a group smoking between 10 and 30 cigarettes and day, and another 1,000 to a group smoking 50 cigarettes a day. A fifth 1,000 would be told to smoke for a period of years and then give up smoking, another group of 1,000 would be told to smoke pipes, while a seventh 1,000 would be instructed to smoke cigars. In other words, our subjects would not be allowed to choose for themselves what to do but would be allocated by the experimenter on a random basis to these various groups. Why is this distinction important? The answer is very simply that the people who elect to smoke might be constitutionally different from the people who elect not to smoke, and that these constitutional differences might also be responsible for the various diseases to which these different groups succumb. Thus there is a possibility that people who are constitutionally predisposed to develop habits of smoking in later life are also constitutionally predisposed to develop and die of lung cancer. There is little doubt that the smoking habit is firmly grounded in hereditary predisposition; it has been demonstrated by studies of identical and fraternal twins that the greater the hereditary similarity of the twins the greater is their concordance in smoking history. We shall see in a later chapter that this general hypothesis, unlikely as it might sound at first, has in fact considerable experimental backing. At the moment, however, let us simply consider it as a possibility, and let us ask if constitutional factors of this kind could indeed be responsible for the facts as reported.

It is with the purpose of illustrating this point that Yerushalmy conducted a series of investigations into the smoking habits of parents and the weights of their children. As his measure for infant weight he used the percentage of babies weighing less than 5 lbs 8 ozs at birth. The main findings are given in Figure 10 which shows a strong association between cigarette smoking of the *father* and the percent of infants wighing less than 5 lbs 8 ozs. Cigarette-smoking fathers tended to have lighter babies than non-cigarette-smoking fathers. This association is clearly a quantitative one, as the more the father smoked the larger was the percentage of infants weighing less than 5 lbs 8 ozs, the percentages ranging from 6·7 for infants whose fathers smoked less than one pack of cigarettes a day, to 10·8 for infants whose fathers smoked more than two packs a day. It will also be seen that infants whose fathers gave up the habit of smoking did not differ in their birth weights from those whose fathers never smoked. Yerushalmy comments that 'The association between cigarette smoking of the father and birth weight of the infant presents therefore a picture very similar to that observed between cigarette smoking and mortality

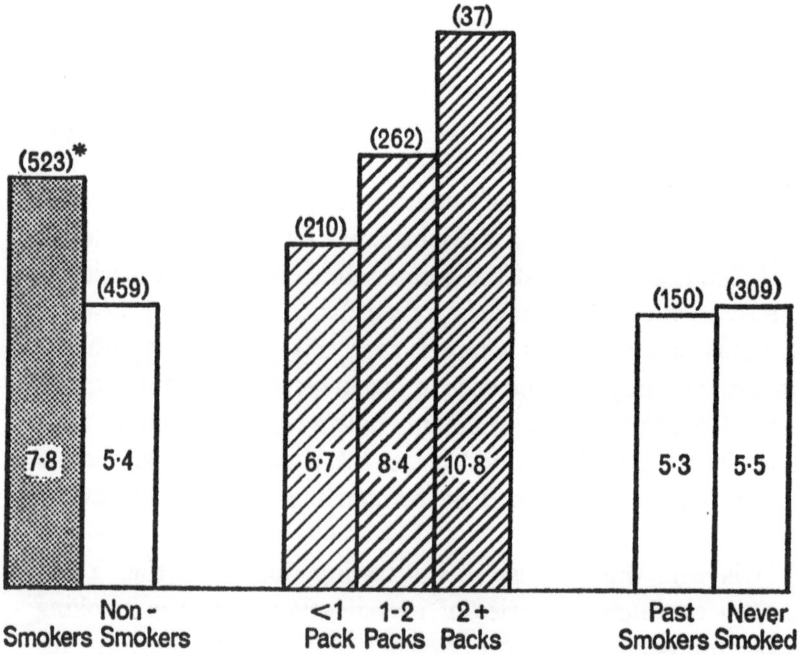

Fig. 10. Per cent of infants weighing less than 5½ lbs according to the cigarette smoking habits of their fathers. Taken with permission from J. Yerushalmy, in 'Tobacco and Health', *op. cit.*, 216.

from a number of diseases. These results, taken by themselves, may be construed as weakening the argument of "specificity" of association between cigarette smoking and mortality of cancer of the lung and other diseases, for while it is possible that the association shown [in Figure 10] indicates a causal relationship few would consider this a strong probability. We are thus again presented with a situation where associations with cigarette smoking are found for a large variety of conditions including one which is not easily acceptable as meaningful in terms of cause and effect.'

Yerushalmy went on to explore the smoking habit of the mother because of the possible association between the smoking habits of husband and wives. A correlation was indeed found between smoking habits of mothers and birth weight of

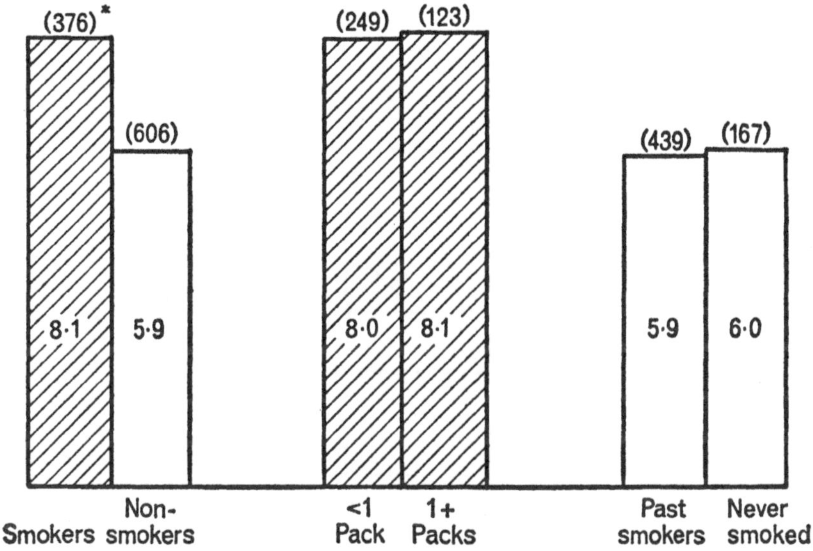

Fig. 11. Per cent of infants weighing less than $5\frac{1}{2}$ lbs according to the cigarette smoking habits of their mothers. Taken with permission from J. Yerushalmy, in 'Tobacco and Health', *op. cit.*, 218.

children and is shown in Figure 11, but it was much weaker for the mother than it was for the father. This odd circumstance led Yerushalmy to investigate the association between birth weight of infant and the smoking habits of both father and mother together and his results are shown in Figure 12.

Yerushalmy comments that 'the striking finding here is that the increase in the percentage of babies weighing less than 5 lbs 8 ozs is present only when the husband and wife both smoke.

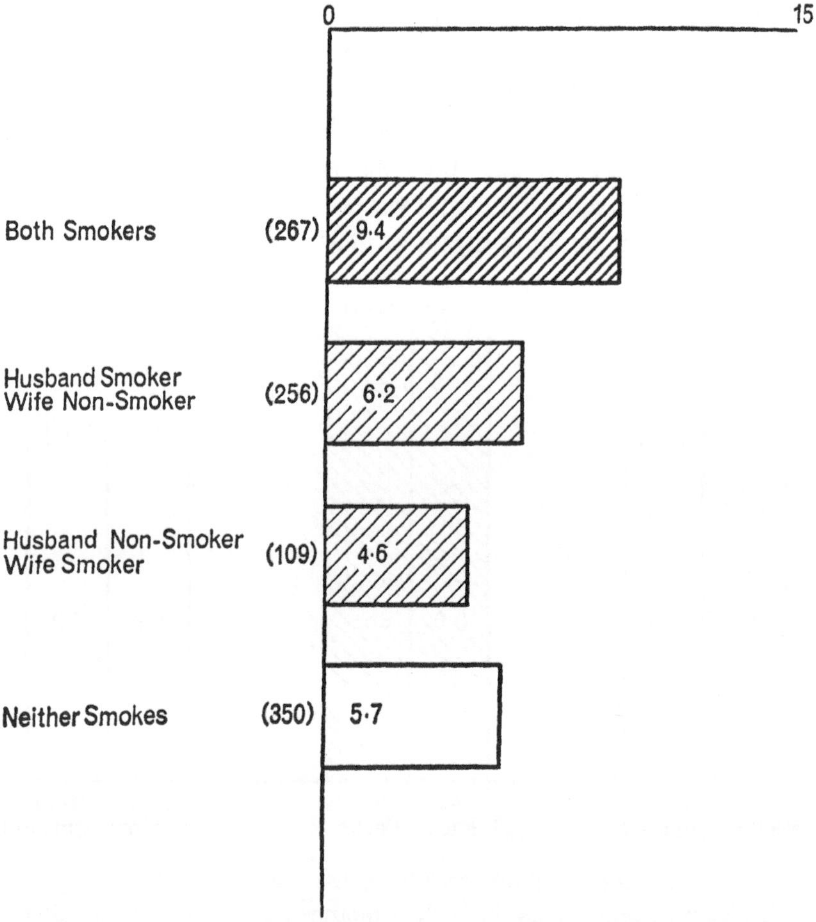

Fig. 12. Per cent of infants weighing less than 5½ lbs according to the cigarette smoking habits of the husband and wife. Taken with permission from J. Yerushalmy, in 'Tobacco and Health', *op. cit.*, 219.

If at least one of them does not smoke – whether it is the husband or the wife – or if neither of them smoke, the proportion of babies under the critical birth weight is approximately the same. There is no difference in the percentages in these three groups of infants. However, the percent weighing less than 5 lbs 8 ozs, both of whose parents smoke, is significantly different from that of infants in the other three groups. Thus it is not that there is an independent father's smoking effect and an independent mother's smoking effect which, when they occur together – both smokers – is more striking. If this were the case the percentage of babies weighing less than 5 lbs 8 ozs would be expected to be much smaller where neither the husband nor the wife smokes. This as may be seen from Figure 12 is not the case. This finding that an increase in the percentage of infants weighing less than 5 lbs 8 ozs is found only when both parents smoke is more difficult to explain on a causal basis than the overall finding of an association with father's smoking habits. It is difficult to visualize a biological mechanism which would exhibit itself in the combined effects of the smoking of both parents, where no effect of smoking of only one of them alone is noted . . . these findings can perhaps more easily be explained on the basis that smoking acts as an index to differentiate smokers from non-smokers on a number of different characteristics rather than as indicating a causal relationship. The lack of 'specificity' which runs through all the associations observed thus far would appear to indicate a strong possibility that smokers differ from non-smokers in many ways including their mode of life and perhaps, as R. A. Fisher suggests, they represent different genotypes. Certainly it provides sufficient cause to question the validity of the argument of causality as the explanation for the association observed between cigarette smoking and lung cancer and the other diseases. At least the lack of 'specificity' weakens the argument for a causal relationship.[15]

Yerushalmy went on to compare the smokers and non-smokers according to a number of other characteristics on which data were available in his study. He found that a larger proportion of fathers who smoked cigarettes also drank coffee, whisky and beer, while relatively more of the non-smokers drank tea, milk and wine. Further, of those who did drink, the average number of cups of coffee per day or of drinks of whisky and beer per week was larger when the father was a smoker than when he was a non-smoker. Similar findings are reported for mothers. It was also found that the fathers who smoked were younger than the non-smoking fathers at the time of birth of their infants in each order of birth.

Yerushalmy concludes: 'In indicating the differences in personality between smokers and non-smokers it is not the intention to suggest that these characteristics are responsible for the increases in mortality from the various diseases or for the decrease in birth weight of the infant. They do, however, bring into sharp focus the fact that the observed differences in mortality according to smoking habits were derived from comparisons of groups that are unlike in many characteristics and consequently great caution must be exercised in interpreting the observed association as proving causality. This is especially true in view of the diffuse association with such a large number of diseases and conditions. We are, therefore, forced either to accept all these associations as indicating a cause/effect relationship or we must find guide lines to determine which of these associations are and which are not meaningful.' Thus the Yerushalmy paradox clearly points out the difficulty which has to be faced by those who maintain the causal theory of the relationship between smoking and lung cancer. Can they suggest any statistical or logical basis on which the lung cancer data are admitted as being causally related to smoking whilst the infant birth weight data are not admitted? To date no such test has been suggested and we remain therefore in the uncomfortable position of either having to assert that there is a causal relationship in the birth weight data, which goes counter to all our biological knowledge of the processes involved, or to admit that there is no evidence of causal relationship in connection with lung cancer.

Quite recently Yerushalmy has added another paradox of a similar kind.[16] It is well known that mothers who smoke during pregnancy have a much larger proportion of their births in the low birth weight group than do mothers who do not smoke. It is also well known that infants of low birth weight have very high neonatal mortality rates. The large excess of infants of low birth weight in mothers who smoke during pregnancy should therefore be accompanied by substantial increase in the neonatal rate of infants of such smoking mothers. Such an increase, however, has never been demonstrated; most investigators find small and insignificant differences between smoking and non-

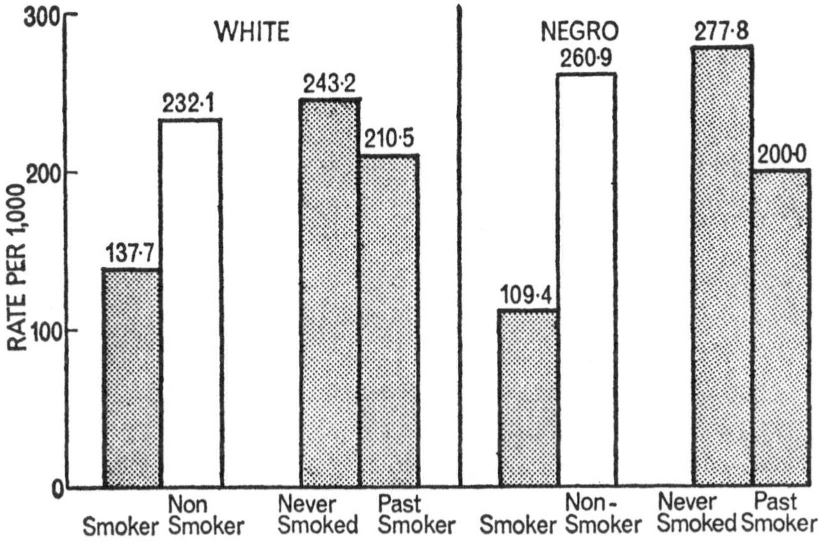

Fig. 13. Neonatal mortality rate per 1,000 for white and negro single live births weighing 5 lb 8 ozs or less according to smoking status of mother. Taken with permission from J. Yerushalmy, *Amer. J. Obst. Gyn.*, 1964, **88**, 511. Published by The C. V. Mosley Company, St.Louis, Missouri.

smoking mothers in the survival of their infants. In a very competent investigation of large numbers of white and negro mothers Yerushalmy investigated the mortality rate for babies weighing 5 lbs 8 ozs or less at birth according to the smoking habits of the mother. The results are given in Figure 13. It will be seen that the mortality rates for both white and negro mothers are significantly greater for non-smoking mothers than for smoking mothers. Equally they are higher for those who never smoked than for those who smoked in the past but gave it up. (The term non-smoker in the figure means mothers who were not smoking at the time of bearing the child; they are subdivided into those who never smoked, and those who did smoke in the past but gave it up before pregnancy.) Thus these figures resolve the original problem; they indicate that mothers who smoke do indeed have smaller infants but that these smaller infants survive more frequently, i.e. have a lower mortality rate than do the children of non-smoking mothers. Again it seems exceedingly unlikely that there should be any causal relationship such as that smoking actually protects the children from the dangers attending any birth. It seems much more likely that here again we are concerned with genetic differences between smokers and non-smokers.

To the Yerushalmy paradox we might perhaps add another one which may be called the Berkson paradox.[17] Berkson compiled a general review of recent death rates by marital status of specific categories of cause of death, dividing people up into married, widowed, single and divorced. His main results for men and women are shown in Figure 14, where it will be seen that for both sexes and at all ages the death rates of the married are lowest and very generally, though not at every age, the death rates among the divorced are the highest, while the rates for the single and widowed lie between. The standardized rates increase in the order, married, single, widowed, divorced. In the rest of his argument Berkson has concentrated on the single, married and divorced groups as the widowed class is less homogeneous and also smaller.

Berkson next considered the death rate from cancer of the lung according to marital state, giving figures separately for the United States as a whole and also for New York State; these are reproduced in Figure 15. It will be seen that the death rates increase among these classes in the order, married, single, divorced, for males and for females, and that this relation is

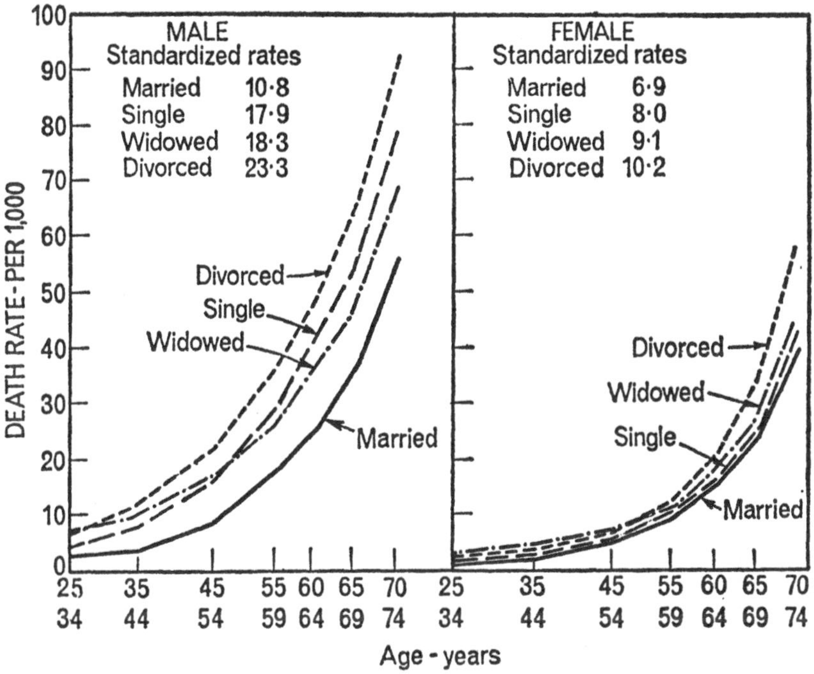

Fig. 14. Death rates from all causes in the United States plotted by marital status. Taken with permission from J. Berkson, *Amer. J. Public Health*, 1962, 52, 1320.

exhibited in both areas studied – the United States as a whole and New York State separately.

Berkson now argues as follows: 'In some analyses of statistical data relating to smoking and cancer of the respiratory organs the conclusion was drawn that smoking is the cause of all deaths from cancer of the lung except possibly a small portion due to air pollution. Were this true, it would follow ineluctably that the increasing death rate from cancer of the lung shown in the figure must be explained by the progressively increasing amount of cigarette smoking in the classes, married,

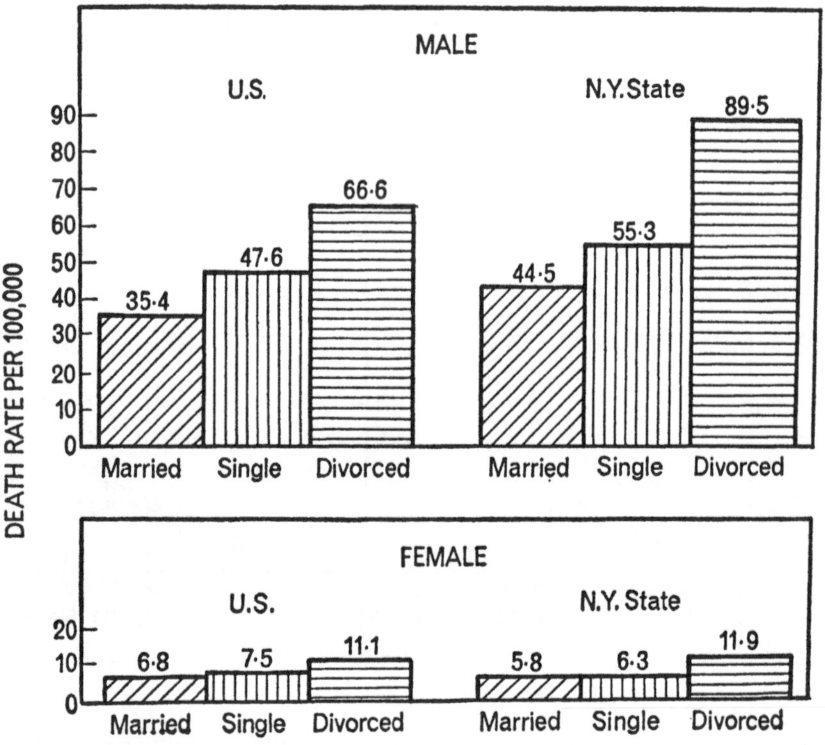

Fig. 15. Death rates for cancer of the respiratory system by marital status given separately for the United States and New York State. Taken with permission from J. Berkson, *Amer. J. Public Health*, 1962, 52, 1324.

single, divorced (except possibly for a small portion due to progressive exposure to polluted air). Now, there do not appear to be any extensive statistics on the relation of smoking to marital status, but published studies indicate that cigarette smoking rates are higher for the married than for the single rather than smaller, and this is in reverse of what is required to explain the low death rate of the married.'

However, detailed examination of figures for other diseases

discloses an even more curious position. As Berkson points out: 'The death rates for the marital classes in the United States increases monotonically in the order, married, single, divorced – and in both sexes – for such diverse disease groups as heart disease and cancer, arteriosclerosis and benign neoplasms, suicide and appendicitis, peptic ulcers and tuberculosis, nephritis, accidents and bronchitis . . . if we confine ourselves to the male we can add diabetes and syphilis, homicide and hyperplastic prostate, pneumonia and cerebral haemorrhage, and cirrhosis of the liver as well.' In other words, just as statistical inquiry shows a complete lack of specificity for the effects of cigarette smoking so similarly marital status shows a complete lack of specificity. Few people would be rash enough to argue that the data on marital status unearthed by Berkson indicate a causal relationship, and he himself would of course not make any such claim. However, if the statistical correlations in the case of smoking are to be taken as indicative of a causal relation, why not those relating to marital status? And how can we explain the contradictory direction of the figures in the case of lung cancer? Clearly, statistical inquiry is beset by many dangers and no simple-minded acceptance of a single set of figures as revealing causal dependence is to be taken seriously.

This brings us to the end of our chapter listing some of the criticisms that have been made of the hypothesis that smoking causes lung cancer and the various other diseases we have mentioned. The reader's state of mind at this point is likely to be one of confusion. Chapter 2 has put a very strong and convincing case in favour of the causal relationship between smoking and lung cancer; Chapter 3 has put an equally cogent and strong case against it. Where does the truth lie? And why is it that in spite of these criticisms so many highly qualified people still believe in the causal hypothesis? The answer probably is, as Conant once pointed out, that theories in science are not overthrown by criticism, however well justified; they are overthrown only by better theories. Until the data summarized in

Chapter 2 can be explained in terms of an alternative theory, so long will the critics be batting on a very poor wicket. It is the main purpose of this book to propose such an alternative theory and to this task we must now turn.

Chapter 4

Personality and Constitution

It is much easier to be critical than correct.

DISRAELI

WE HAVE ALREADY referred several times to the so-called constitutional theory of lung cancer and smoking, i.e. the hypothesis first put forward by Sir Ronald Fisher that people of a certain constitutional type are particularly prone to lung cancer and are also particularly predisposed to take up cigarette smoking. In this form the theory is too weak to be very useful because it is so indefinite that no specific test can be conducted to support or disprove it. What is maintained in effect is that there are certain types of people who smoke; that this type of person has acquired his particular personality through hereditary causes, and that this particular type of person is also more likely to develop cancer. Clearly, therefore, psychological studies are needed to link up both smoking and cancer proneness with specific personality types. It is the purpose of the present chapter to demonstrate such a link between personality and smoking, but in order to do so we must first of all consider very briefly the description and measurement of personality.

The concept of personality in psychology is a very confused one and the term is used by many different people in many different ways.[18] Essentially, however, there are two main definitions or ways of looking at personality. The first of these may be called the behaviouristic view. As an example of this approach we may quote J. B. Watson, the originator of behaviourism. According to him personality is: 'The sum of activities that can be discovered by actual observation over a long enough period of time to give reliable information.' It will be seen that this definition deals entirely with observable behaviour patterns, and personality is defined in terms of such patterns. Such a definition has obvious advantages. The term 'personality' is removed from the almost mystical aura which surrounds it in the writings of so many people and planted firmly and squarely in the realm of observable data.

A quite different way of looking at personality is the so-called dynamic or psychoanalytic approach. The views of Freud, Jung, Adler and other well-known analysts deal almost entirely with hypothetical and unconscious causes supposedly underlying behaviour, such as the Oedipus complex, Electra complex and so forth. In their view actual behaviour is relatively unimportant; what is important are the unconscious roots of behaviour which can only be discovered through psychoanalytic interpretation of dreams and other sources of data of a rather non-behavioural type. In this chapter we will deal exclusively with the behaviouristic type of approach. There are several reasons for this. In the first place, practically all the experimental work which is available to us has been done from this point of view. In the second place, the evidence for the hypothetical 'dynamic' determinants of behaviour is so scant, unscientific and ambiguous that little or no reliance can be placed on it. It cannot be the purpose of this chapter to go into any detail in respect to these points; the reader who is inclined to pursue this point further is referred to some of the references given in this chapter.[19]

How shall we set about describing personality? We have two time-hallowed methods of discovering details about that type of behaviour which we have agreed to subsume under the title of 'personality': one is the method of observation in which we rate the person for his degree of sociability, persistence, suggestibility or whatever trait we might be interested in. The second method is one in which we ask him questions such as whether he likes going to parties, whether he tends to plan things well in advance or whether he likes to play pranks on other people. From the answers to a long list of carefully selected questions surprisingly detailed and accurate information may be obtained about a person's habitual behaviour patterns. A third and more recent method of studying personality is the experimental method. Here we make up tests in the laboratory and measure the responses of our subjects on these tests. All three methods, of course, have their difficulties and are subject to criticism. However, these criticisms are all rather different and when we find that all three methods agree in a given case then we can have some confidence that the results are indeed correct.[20]

The oldest and still very popular method of describing personality was in terms of types. Everyone has heard of the four temperaments originally put forward by Hippocrates and later made popular in Europe by Galen, a Greek physician who lived in the second century of our era. According to their view there were four main types: the melancholic, the choleric, the sanguine and the phlegmatic. It used to be believed until quite recently that every person belonged to one of these four types, and that no intermediate types were possible and no mixing of types could take place. Figure 16 in the inner circle shows the position as described by Galen. The theory fell into disrepute because, quite clearly, although *some* people were described very accurately by these terms the majority of people did not resemble any one of them very closely but tended to be intermediate. The position is rather as if we tended to call all people either tall or short; this agrees to some extent with reality but is rather too restrictive. We are much better off by recognizing a scale of measurement according to which we measure people's height in inches or in centimetres. Even if we added a third group to the tall and short groups, i.e. an average or intermediate group, it will still be clear that proper measurement along a continuum is preferable to the allocation of everybody to one of a limited and rather small number of types.

How can we translate a categorical system involving four quite separate categories or types into one using continuous measurement? The first to suggest the correct answer was the famous German psychologist Wilhelm Wundt. He pointed out that the

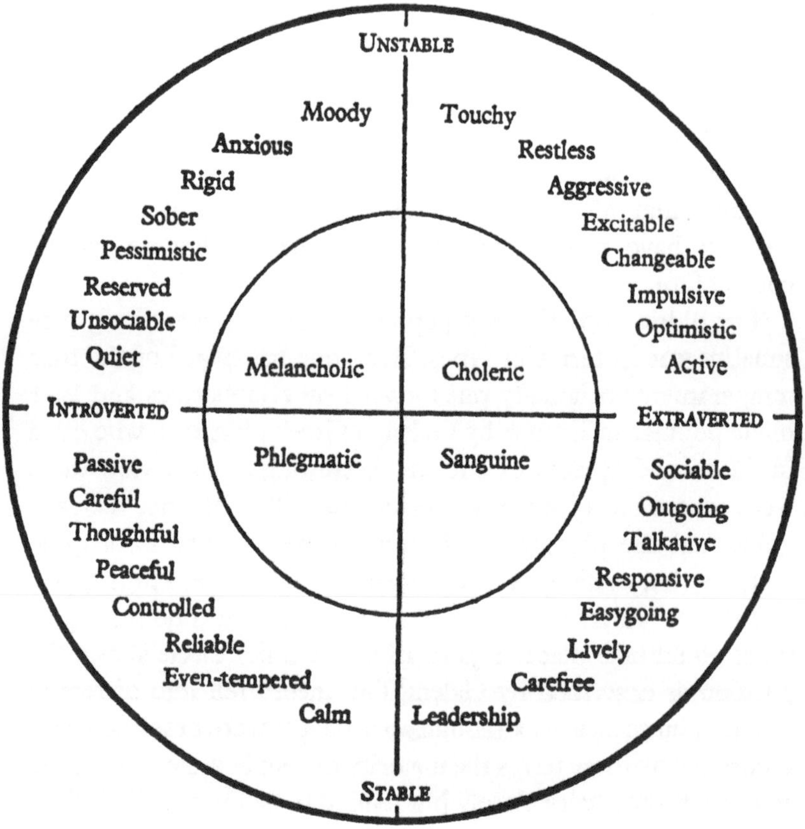

Fig. 16. Diagrammatic view of descriptive system of personality. Inner circle shows the 'four temperaments'; outer circle shows patterning of personality traits according to modern research. Taken from H. J. Eysenck, 'Crime and Personality', 1964.

melancholics and the cholerics were alike in showing very strong emotional reactions, whereas the phlegmatics and the sanguines were alike in showing rather weak emotional reactions. Consequently, he suggested the existence of a dimension or continuum of *strong* as opposed to *weak* emotionality. Similarly, he thought that cholerics and sanguines tended to have emotions which were rather changeable, whereas melancholics and phlegmatics tended to have emotions which were rather firm and stable. Thus he transformed a system of four independent types into one of two independent dimensions, labelled emotionality and changeability. A given person might be assigned any position from one extreme through the centre to the other extreme on either of these two dimensions, and it was a combination of positions on these two dimensions which produced his 'temperament'. A person with strong emotions and also very changeable would then be a choleric, a person with weak emotions but stable would be a phlegmatic and so on. All possible combinations were capable of occurring and there was no question of fixed unchanging categories.

The dimension which Wundt called strong as opposed to weak emotionality is still frequently called 'emotionality' by psychologists, but is also sometimes referred to as 'neuroticism' because by and large strong emotions tend to produce very frequently neurotic disturbances. The dimension of 'changeable' as opposed to 'unchangeable' is now frequently called extraversion as opposed to introversion. In our figure we have used these terms, 'introverted' and 'extraverted', to denote this dimension and we have called the other 'unstable' as opposed to 'stable'. The precise nature of these dimensions can be understood best by reference to the trait names in the outer circle. These are the results of large-scale empirical investigations into the relations between traits in a great variety of different types of people of different social classes, different races and different nationalities. All these studies, whether carried out in England, America, the European continent, Japan, India or Arabia, give results indicating that the unstable end of the emotionality continuum is characterized by moodiness, touchiness, restlessness, anxiety, rigidity, aggressiveness and so forth, whereas the stable end is characterized by calmness, carefreeness, liveliness, reliability and an even temper.

How about extraversion and introversion? Here we will give a more detailed description because we are going to use these terms rather freely in this chapter. According to empirical studies then the typical extravert is sociable, likes parties, has many friends, needs to have people to talk to, and does not like reading or studying by himself; he craves excitement, takes chances, acts on the spur of the moment and is generally an impulsive individual. He is fond of practical jokes, always has a ready answer and generally likes change; he is carefree, easy-going, optimistic and likes to 'laugh and be merry'. He prefers to keep moving and doing things, tends to be aggressive and loses his temper quickly; his feelings are not kept under tight control and he is not always a reliable person.

The typical introvert on the other hand is a quiet, retiring sort of person, introspective, fond of books rather than people; he is reserved and reticent except with intimate friends. He tends to plan ahead, 'looks before he leaps' and distrusts the impulse of the moment. He does not like excitement, takes matters of everyday life with proper seriousness and likes a well ordered mode of life. He keeps his feelings under close control, seldom behaves in an aggressive manner and does not lose his temper easily. He is reliable, somewhat pessimistic and places great value on ethical standards.

The reader will have noted the close similarity between the original descriptions of Hippocrates and Galen and the more modern descriptions given above based on empirical data, and he may have wondered how these data were in fact derived. In essence what is done is to present a large number of subjects with a personality questionnaire or inventory which contains questions relevant to the personality traits the investigator is interested in. Having obtained answers to these questions he then assesses the degree of similarity between any two traits by a mathematical technique known as correlation. If two traits are practically always found together in the same people then the correlation will be very high, approximating unity. If there is no particular relation between two traits so that knowing that a person possesses trait 1 does not tell us anything about whether he does or does not possess trait 2 the correlation will be zero. If nearly everyone who possesses trait A does not possess trait B then the correlation will be negative and approximate unity. We can go on to analyse the pattern of interrelations so disclosed and discover something very much like the picture disclosed in Figure 17. Here the numbers refer to the questions in the questionnaire and their relative positions indicate the degree of correlation; the closer two numbers are together the closer is the relationship within the population studied of the two traits concerned. Thus our dimension of extraversion will be seen to be made up largely of four traits, sociability, liveliness, jocularity and impulsiveness. Consider sociability. This is defined by a number of questions such as the one labelled 37 which goes: 'Do you usually stay in the background at parties and get-togethers?' (The r after the number 37 in Figure 17 indicates that 'no' is the answer indicative of sociability.) Similarly question 29 reads: 'Generally, do you prefer reading to meeting people?', whereas question 93 goes like this: 'Do you find it hard to really enjoy yourself at a lively party?' Question 95 reads: 'Do you usually keep yourself to yourself except with very close friends?' And lastly question 49 reads: 'Can you usually let yourself go and enjoy yourself a lot at a gay party?'

The trait of jocularity is represented by three questions. One is number 53: 'Do you like practical jokes?' The second is 77: 'Do you hate being with a crowd who play jokes on one another?'; here of course the answer no is the one indicative of jocularity. Lastly we have 101: 'Do you like playing pranks on others?'

Just one last example from the other factor here labelled neuroticism. Consider the trait called 'sensitivity' which is defined by three questions. These are first of all 26: 'Are your feelings rather easily hurt?' Next 82: 'Does it bother you to have people watch you work?' And lastly number 90: 'Are you easily hurt when people find fault with you or your work?' These few illustrations of course cannot suffice to give the

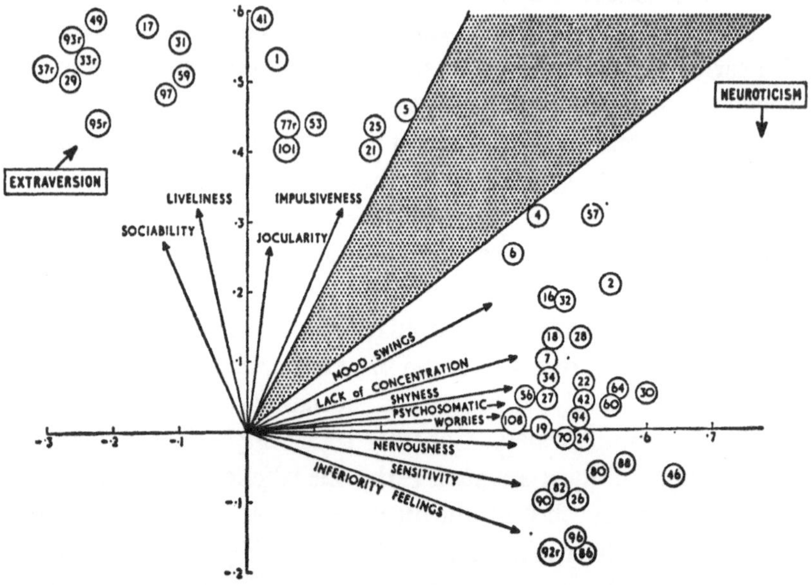

Fig. 17. Diagram illustrating the way in which the two main dimensions of personality are made up of clusters of traits. For explanation, see text.

reader much of an impression of the type of work that is being done with questionnaires, but there is no room for any further elaboration. Suffice it that a great deal of careful and highly technical work goes into the preparation of questionnaires; they are not just hastily thrown together lists of arbitrary questions but are the end results of over 50 years of statistical examination of relationships between different types of questions in very many different types of populations.

Are questionnaires like this valid? In other words, when people answer a questionnaire of this kind in an extraverted or introverted manner is their behaviour really accurately represented by their replies? The answer to this must be that on the whole the resemblance is remarkably close. This answer has to be qualified by insisting that a truthful description of a person's temperament can only be obtained when he is not motivated in any way to represent himself in a more favourable light. It would be useless for instance to give questionnaires like this to people applying for a job because obviously they would argue that their obtaining the job would depend on the answers, and that they would be quite justified in putting themselves in the best light. That this is so has indeed been shown experimentally. A questionnaire was given to a large number of applicants for a particular type of job; half the applicants were given the questionnaire *before* the decision was made of hiring them or not, the other half were given the questionnaire *after* they had been engaged. It was found that those who answered the questionnaire while still in doubt whether they would be hired or not gave answers which were much more favourable to themselves than did those who had already been hired, and for whom therefore the filling of the questionnaire was merely an academic exercise. This, of course, is not surprising and it would be unreasonable to expect any other outcome. However, under ordinary conditions where a person is co-operating in an experiment, it has been found that replies are remarkably truthful. Consider just two items of evidence. When normal people and neurotic patients are given personality questionnaires there is usually hardly any overlap at all between them with respect to the neuroticism factor: the neurotics have very high emotional scores whereas the normals have very much smaller ones. Similarly, when groups of judges pick out from among people known to them extreme extraverts and extreme introverts as judged in terms of their behaviour, and when these extreme introverts and extraverts are then administered questionnaires, it is found that there is very high agreement between the judges and the scores of the persons designated by them. Those designated as extraverts do give extraverted scores, those designated as introverts give introverted scores. There is thus sufficient reliability and validity to questionnaire measurement of personality under experimental conditions to make it useful and valuable.

The majority of people of course are neither particularly introverted nor particularly extraverted, neither particularly stable nor particularly neurotic. One would expect, however, that those who have scores tending towards the extremes would show behaviour patterns which would make them sufficiently outstanding to be socially noticed. That this is true is shown in Figure 18. This figure gives in diagrammatic form the scores on questionnaires of extraversion/introversion and of neuroticism, of neurotic patients and of criminals in prison. It will be seen that the neurotics are strongly introverted as well as high on neuroticism (emotionality), whereas the prisoners are high on extraversion and equally high on neuroticism (emotionality) as are the neurotics. Thus there is good external evidence to show that individuals having certain types of scores on these personality questionnaires do in fact differ from each other very markedly with respect to personality patterns, which brings them into contact with psychiatrist and mental hospitals in the case of the people in the 'melancholic' quadrant, and with courts and prisons in the case of the people in our 'choleric' quadrant. These results are predictable in terms of the theory of personality described in our next chapter and readers who may be interested in the application of that theory to these two fields are referred to the author's book *Crime and Personality*[21] which deals with the emotional extraverts, and to *Causes and Cures of Neurosis* by the present writer and Dr S. Rachman,[22] which deals with the emotional introvert.

There are, of course, very many other observable behaviour patterns which discriminate the extravert from the introvert. Extraverts change their jobs more frequently and also their marriage partners; in addition they are more likely to have premarital and extra-marital intercourse. Unmarried mothers tend to be predominantly extraverted, as indicated in Figure 18. Extraverts drink more alcohol than do introverts, and they prefer spicy foods more frequently. They are more likely to have driving accidents and to be booked for driving offences. Introverts do better at academic work than do extraverts.

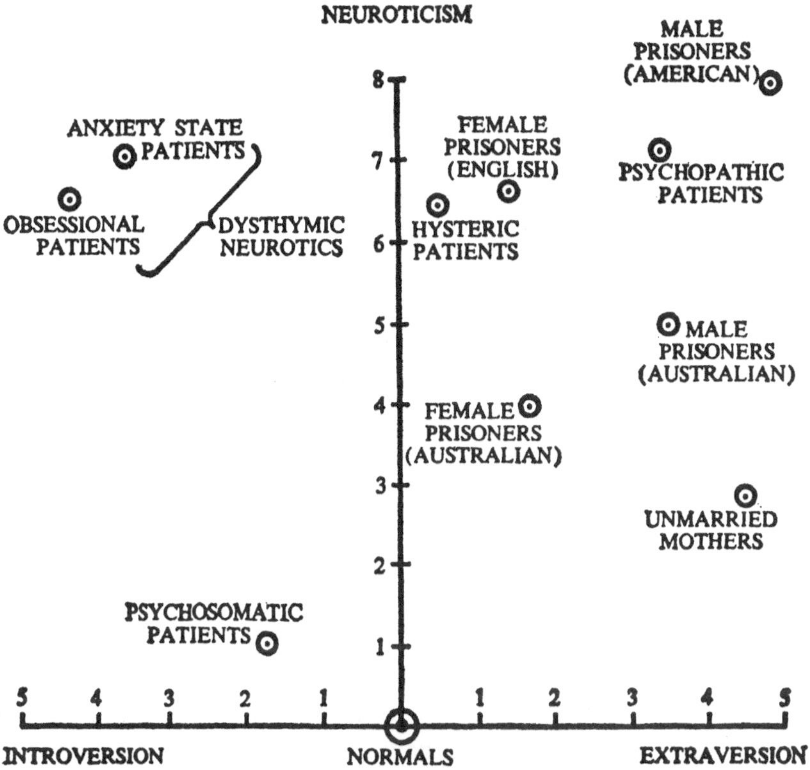

Fig. 18. Diagram showing the position of neurotics and criminals with respect to two main dimensions of personality. Both groups are high on neuroticism (emotionality), but where neurotics are introverted, criminals are extraverted. Taken from H. J. Eysenck 'Crime and Personality', 1964.

Introverts tend to be more 'self-directed', extraverts more 'other-directed'. These are just some of the findings in this field but they may suffice to give the reader an idea of the range of social situations to which this concept of extraversion/introversion applies.

We now have two main dimensions of personality which can be measured with reasonable accuracy and which we will find useful in our discussion of the relationship between personality and smoking. It need hardly be said that these two dimensions do not make up the whole of human personality. All that needs to be said is that they cover some important and relevent aspects of our inquiry; no greater claim than that is made for them. Let it also be noted that they are used in a purely descriptive manner. Clearly, it would be quite wrong to say that a person behaved in a sociable manner or an impulsive manner because he possessed a trait of sociability or impulsiveness, when our only evidence for these hypothetical traits is the fact that he did behave in the past in a sociable or impulsive manner! Descriptively, therefore, dimensions derived in this statistical manner from known behaviour in the past are useful and scientifically acceptable; they do require further support, however, from some kind of causal theory such as that discussed in the next chapter.

For the moment, however, we must investigate another question that is more immediately relevant to our main inquiry, and that is the dependence of these main personality dimensions on hereditary and constitutional factors. Most of the studies carried out in this field have made use of identical and fraternal twins. The first to point out the value of twins for the study of genetic influence was Sir Francis Galton, a cousin of Charles Darwin, who was born in 1822. It was already known in his time that there were two different types of twins. In the case of identical twins there is one sperm uniting with one ovum which later on, after fertilization has taken place, breaks in two, thus giving rise to two separate and independent individuals; these are always of the same sex and share identical heredity. In the other type of twin, the so-called fraternal or heterozygotic type, two ova are fertilized simultaneously by two sperms and the two individuals that result are no more alike than ordinary brothers and sisters. They need not be identical with respect to sex and are so only in half the cases. Galton noted that many twins of the same sex were alike from birth, and tended to remain alike in their height and girth, their behaviour, their temperament and even in the diseases to which they fell prey. Twins of unlike sex, however, tended to be much more unlike each other in these respects as were a proportion of like sex twins. Galton's fundamental theoretical work in this field has been fully confirmed since and nowadays it is quite easy to diagnose a given pair of twins as identical or fraternal. This is usually done by looking for similarities or differences in respect to certain features which are known to be inherited, such as blood group, finger prints and so forth. When these are concongruous, probability is high that the twins are identical; when they are different it is practically certain that the twins are not identical but fraternal.

How can we use the existence of this sport of nature in an investigation of the inheritance of a given trait or ability? Let us take a trait which is determined entirely by environmental influences, and let us compare groups of identical and groups of fraternal twins. As heredity plays no part in the determination of individual differences in this trait the fact that identical twins have identical heredity does not make them any more alike than our fraternal twins, and therefore we shall find no greater differences between fraternal twins than we do between identical twins. The situation, however, should be quite different if we took a trait which was determined in its manifestations to a considerable extent by hereditary influences. Here the identical heredity of the identical twins should make them much more alike than the fraternal twins, and the observed differences between the two groups should give us a very good indication of the importance to be attached to the hereditary influences at work. This is the rationale underlying the use of the twin method in this type of research and has been very widely used indeed.

What happens when we measure the extraversion or the degree of neuroticism of identical and fraternal twins and compare these two groups with each other? The experiment has been done a number of times using both questionnaires and objective laboratory tests and the outcome has been very similar in each case. With regard to both extraversion and neuroticism identical twins are very much more alike than are fraternal twins, and this seems to indicate that heredity plays a very strong part in the causation of individual differences in these two dimensions of personality. While it is impossible to give a very accurate assessment it may be said that in our type of culture and under ordinary conditions of upbringing heredity accounts for something like three-quarters of the individual differences in extraversion or neuroticism which we observe in the population. This is very similar in degree to the determination of intelligence by hereditary factors, and it indicates very strongly that our hypothesis of constitutional factors in the determination of behaviour may have been along the correct lines.

There is one criticism which is sometimes made of these studies and it goes like this. It is said that perhaps identical twins are treated more alike by parents, teachers and other children and that consequently they develop more similar personality patterns; fraternal twins, on the same argument, would not be treated as much in the same sort of way and consequently would develop along somewhat more different lines. This argument may sound plausible, although direct observation of the way identical and fraternal twins are treated does not support it; usually parents and teachers and other children are quite unaware of the differences between identical and fraternal twins and simply regard them as twins. However, more important than such theoretical consideration is a recent experiment performed by Dr James Shields of the Maudsley Hospital. [23] In it he compared three groups with respect to intelligence, extraversion and neuroticism. One group was made up of fraternal twins, the second group was made up of identical twins brought up together, and the third group was made up of identical twins brought up in separation from an early age. He found that fraternal were much less alike than identical twins, but, he also found that identical twins brought up together were slightly less alike than were identical twins brought up in separation! This finding would seem to disprove conclusively this common objection to the use of twins in research of this kind. It is interesting to note that the finding was identical for all three measures, i.e. intelligence, extraversion and neuroticism.

At the end of this chapter, then, we arrive at the conclusion that there are two very important, wide-ranging dimensions of personality which are based on hereditary factors and which can be measured with reasonable accuracy by means of questionnaires and objective experimental tests. If we could show that smoking was related to one or both of these dimensions and if we could show additionally that the development of cancer and perhaps coronary disease was also related to the same dimension or dimensions then we would have found some support for the constitutional hypothesis. The next chapter will discuss some of the evidence relating to both these points.

Chapter 5

Smokers and Non-Smokers

And the smoke of their torment ascendeth up for ever and ever; and they have no rest day or night, who worship the beast and his image.

HOLY BIBLE

THE FACT THAT individual differences in the two main dimensions of personality are largely determined by heredity suggests very strongly that these dimensions of personality must depend on some physiological or neurological structures. The reason for this hypothesis is, of course, that it is conceivable that such structures should be transmitted through the physical action of the genes and chromosomes which carry hereditary information, but that it is not conceivable that behaviour patterns as such should be transmitted in this way without any reference to biological structures. Is there any evidence for a relationship between personality patterns and physiological structures?

As far as neuroticism is concerned the answer is quite simple. It will be recalled that an alternative name for neuroticism which was first used by Wundt and has since been used by many others too is 'emotionality'. In other words, people who have a high score on tests of neuroticism tend to be people who have labile emotions, that is to say emotions that are easily aroused and which persist much longer than would be customary in the average person. Now there is a particular part of our nervous system which deals predominantly with the expression of the emotions. This is the so-called autonomic system which derives its name from the fact that it is partly at least independent of the central nervous system. The central nervous system is mainly concerned with perception, that is to say the transmission of impulses from eyes, ears, nose, the skin and other receptor areas to the cortex, and with voluntary activity, i.e. the innervation of muscles which gives rise to movement. The autonomic system is concerned with a large variety of behaviour patterns which are largely unconscious and not under the control of the will. The beating of the heart for instance, breathing, particularly when we are asleep, changes in the electric conductivity of the skin subsequent to the stimulation of the sweat glands – these and many other responses are mediated by the autonomic system. This system itself is divided into two antagonistic parts, the so-called sympathetic and the parasympathetic. The sympathetic is the part of the autonomic which governs our 'fight or flight' reactions; in other words, it makes the body ready for energetic activity. It speeds up the heart beat and the rate of breathing in order to make available more blood and oxygen to the body; it produces an increase in the size of the pupil of the eye in order to admit more light so that we can see better for the purpose of either running away or fighting; it stops digestion in order to make the blood available for more immediately necessary activities. Most of these activities we are quite unconscious of, some of them we do experience quite consciously although probably more in recollection than at the actual time. Thus if the reader has ever been very much afraid, or very angry, he may recall the beating of the heart, the rapid breathing, the drying out of the mouth and other similar bodily effects which are mediated by the sympathetic system. The parasympathetic on the other hand, while acting on the same bodily structures, has an action which is the exact opposite to that of the sympathetic. The parasympathetic slows the heart, slows down breathing, improves digestion and generally is conducive to a peaceful, vegetating existence.

It is this autonomic system which is closely related to the personality structure of neuroticism as opposed to stability.

What characterizes the neurotic is a highly labile autonomic system which is aroused too easily, and remains in a state of arousal much too long. There is evidence that individual differences in autonomic reactivity are indeed largely inherited and some interesting work has been carried out on rats with the aim of breeding strains which should be particularly emotional or non-emotional. The test used in these studies was the so-called open field test in which a rat is put into a circular enclosure, brightly illuminated and kept at a high noise level by loudspeakers. The rats are frightened and react by urinating and depositing fecal bolusses in the enclosure. The number of these fecal bolusses deposited is the score and it is notable that some individuals deposit hardly any at all, while others deposit quite a few. We can now pick out the reactive animals who deposit a large number of fecal bolusses and interbreed them; in the next generation we again pick out the most reactive animals and interbreed them, and so on for several generations in turn.

Similarly for the non-reactive group, we pick out those who deposit the smallest number of bolusses, interbreed them and go on from each successive generation to pick out the least reactive animals and interbreed them in turn. Figure 19 illustrates the results of such an experiment carried out in our laboratories for fifteen generations.[24] It will be seen that at the beginning three bolusses were deposited on the average by the original parent generation during the length of the test. The reactive animals bred selectively finally had a mean score of 4 bolusses whereas the non-reactive animals had a mean score of zero. There was practically no overlap between the two pure-bred strains and a great deal of knowledge is now available about the precise mode of inheritance of this general trait of emotionality or reactivity.

It should not be imagined that we are dealing here only with a very limited habit which is inherited, to wit the deposition of a certain number of fecal bolusses in a particular stressful situation. Reactive and non-reactive rats differ on a large number of experimental tests in which emotion is aroused and determines

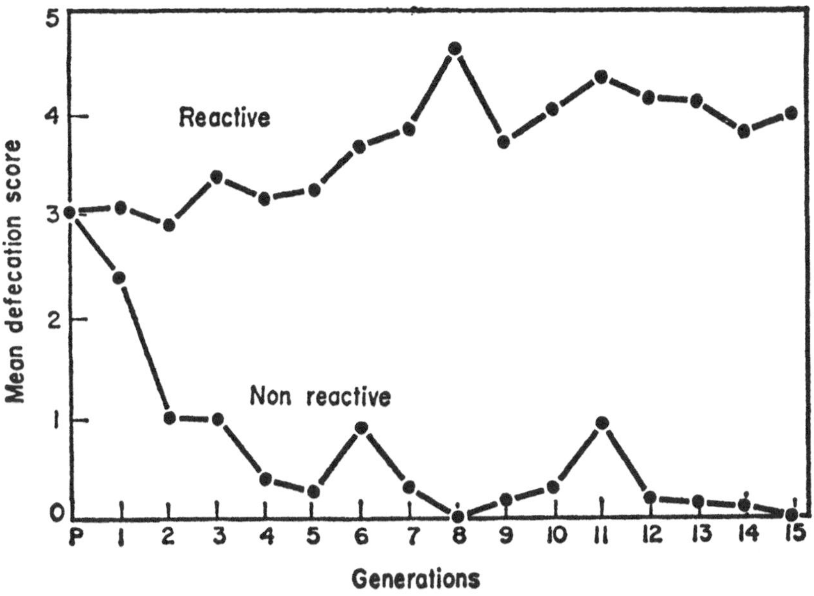

Fig. 19. Scores on a test of emotionality of 15 generations of rats bred for their emotional reactivity or lack of reactivity, respectively. For explanation, see text. Taken from a chapter by P. L. Broadhurst, in H. J. Eysenck 'Experiments in Personality', 1960.

behaviour, and it is predictable in each case how the two groups will react. We thus have here an animal analogue of human emotionality inherited along very similar lines and mediated by the autonomic system and by secretions from some of the well-known endocrine glands. While many details remain to be discovered the general outline of the physiological basis for our dimension of emotionality or neuroticism seems to be fairly clear.

How about extraversion and introversion? Here use may be made of two concepts, which were originally suggested by the great Russian physiologist, I. Pavlov, namely the concepts of excitation and inhibition. What is meant by excitation here is essentially a facilitative action of the cortex in mediating perception, attention and mental work generally; inhibition means the opposite, i.e. interference with the on-going work of the brain. A brain in a high state of excitation is optimally qualified to deal with incoming information from the outer world and react appropriately; the brain in a state of inhibition is less well qualified to cope. Cortical excitation and inhibition may themselves be the product of sub-cortical activity particularly in the so-called ascending reticular formation. This sub-cortical structure receives impulses from the long afferent pathways which lead from the periphery of the body to the brain, and in turn bombards the cortex with impulses. Some of these impulses are of an 'activating' nature, i.e. they keep the cortex in a high state of excitation and efficiency and without them the effect of incoming impulses would be momentary and would soon give rise to periods of drowsiness or sleep. There is also, however, part of the ascending reticular formation, the so-called recruiting or synchronizing part, which has the opposite effect, i.e. it inhibits the activity of the cortex. Which of these two parts of the reticular formation is excited depends in part on the nature of the signal. Thus repetitive signals tend to activate the synchronizing part and to lead to inhibition of the cortical activity consequent upon this signal.

The writer has put forward the hypothesis that extraverts are characterized by inhibitory activity in the cortex whereas introverts are characterized by excitatory activity in the cortex.[25] There is much evidence on the physiological level that this hypothesis is true. For instance, we may take tracings of the electrical activity of the brain through the so-called electroencephalograph; prominent in such tracings is the so-called alpha rhythm, a rhythmic activity of some 10 cycles per second which is particularly noticeable under conditions of drowsiness and when the subject closes his eyes, i.e. when there is a certain amount of synchronization or inhibition observable in the cortex. According to our theory such alpha activity should be much more prominent in extraverts than in introverts and this has indeed been found to be so. There is much other evidence of a similar kind, but as this book is not particularly concerned with physiological details of this kind, we shall not go into them to any greater extent. Let us merely note that the evidence, while far from conclusive, does seem to support some such generalization as that here presented.

Extraverted and introverted behaviour patterns of the kind considered may be due in large part to the inherited characteristics of the cortical and sub-cortical functionings of the individuals, particularly of the reticular formation. But these in turn are not completely incapable of being influenced in certain ways. The most obvious way in which we can in part change the functioning of these structures is by drugs. There are two types of drugs, the so-called *central nervous system stimulant* and *depressant* drugs which are relevant in this context. Depressant drugs like alcohol and the barbiturates have an *inhibitory* action on the cortex and should therefore in terms of our theory lead to a greater degree of extraversion; that that is true, at least as far as alcohol is concerned, is only too well known! Stimulant drugs like caffeine and amphetamine have an *excitatory* effect on the brain and should therefore lead to more introverted behaviour patterns. Many experimental studies have been done along these lines and they have indeed established that broadly speaking this generalization is true. In other words, stimulant drugs lead to introverted behaviour, depressant drugs lead to extraverted behaviour. We may consider for a moment the effect of nicotine which after all is the drug most involved in the smoking of tobacco.[26]

The general literature suggests that nicotine is a stimulant drug. In terms of our theory it should thus produce introverted behaviour patterns. How can we prove such a statement? We must first of all have a test which theoretically measures the degree of excitation or inhibition of the cortex and which additionally has been shown in the past to be responsive to differences between extraverts and introverts. Such a test is the so-called critical flicker fusion test. In this the subject is presented with a flickering light; this is arranged in such a way that the speed with which it flickers, i.e. the number of cycles per second, can be changed in an upward or downward direction. The threshold is the point at which the subject ceases to see the light as flickering and reports that it seems to be still. Now the ability to discriminate the several pulses is dependent on the efficient functioning of the cortex; in other words, a proper degree of activation or excitation is required, and consequently we would expect introverts to have a higher threshold than extraverts, i.e. be able to discriminate the flickering nature of the light after extraverts had ceased to be able to do so. That this is true has been shown in a number of studies and we may therefore accept the c.f.f. test, as it is called, as a suitable one for our purpose.

In one experiment 3 groups of 5 subjects each were tested, one receiving 0·1 mg of nicotine, the second receiving no drugs, and the third receiving a placebo, i.e. dummy tablet which had no effect on the organism at all.[27] The c.f.f. was tested every 5 minutes and the results of the experiment are shown in Figure 20. It will be seen that just preceding the administration of the drug all three groups were very close together having a threshold of about 41 cycles per second; in other words when the light was flashing on and off at the rate of 41 flashes per second the members of all three groups just ceased to see the light as flickering. It will also be seen that the no-drug and the placebo groups continued at this level during the next 20 minutes, but that the group which had received the nicotine went up to almost a rate of 44 cycles per second. In other words, there is a clear-cut effect of the drug in the predicted direction making the cortex more efficient in discriminating the stimuli presented to it. This, of course, is only one typical experiment to illustrate the type of reasoning employed, but others have been carried out with very much the same results. We may conclude, therefore, that nicotine is a stimulant drug and therefore has introverting effects.

How would we expect personality to be related to smoking?

The writer has suggested that on theoretical grounds we would expect extraverts to smoke cigarettes more than would introverts, and it may be of some interest to repeat here the theoretical argument which led to this prediction.[28] Consider first of all Figure 21. This Figure presents a very well-known generaliza-

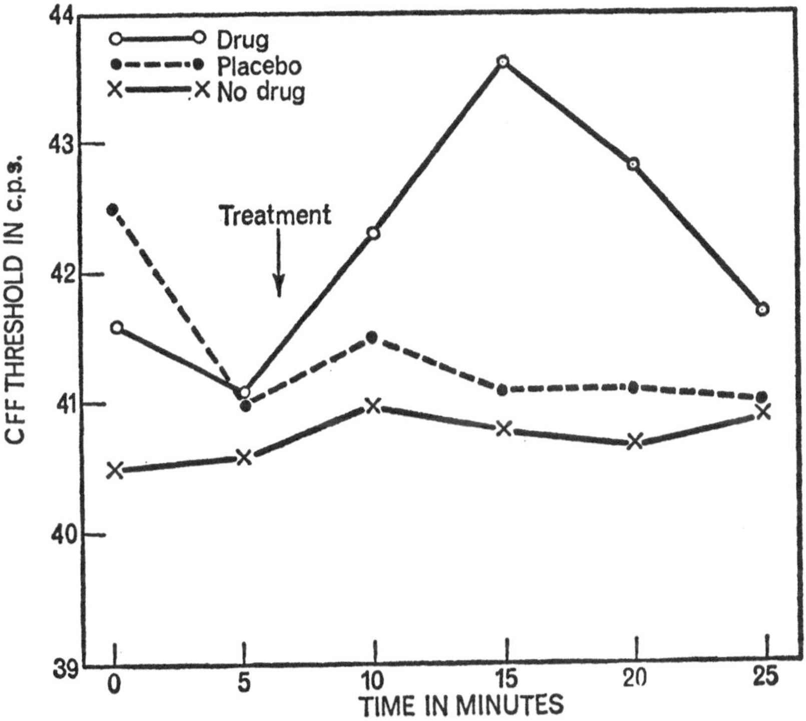

Fig. 20. Critical flicker fusion thresholds under drug, placebo, and no drug conditions. Note the improvement in threshold after administration of nicotine and its subsequent decline as the drug wears off.

tion from many hundreds of studies that have been carried out during the last 100 years relating the *intensity* of stimulation to its *hedonic effects*, i.e. the liking or disliking of the effect by the person experiencing it. The relationship is indicated by the thick curved line in the centre of the diagram, and it will be seen that there is a tendency for very strong stimulation to give rise to negative hedonic tone, i.e. to dislike. Similarly, very weak stimulation, or sensory deprivation as it is sometimes called, also gives rise to a negative hedonic tone, i.e. to dislike. This fact has been established many times, particularly in recent years, where work on sensory deprivation has been carried on very vigorously in view of the possible effects this may have on astronauts during their flight to the moon. In this type of experiment a person is isolated in a room; he wears goggles which do not permit him to discern any details in his surroundings; all sources of auditory stimulation are removed, and in addition he wears cardboard covers over his hands and feet which make it impossible for him to touch anything. Under these conditions subjects who are highly paid to remain in the chamber as long as possible become extremely distressed and may ask to be released after relative short periods. The greater the efficacy of the deprivation the shorter the period during which the subject will tolerate the situation. In other words, both very strong stimulation producing pain and very weak stimulation producing sensory deprivations are equally obnoxious to typical human subjects. There is a very marked preference for intermediate degrees of stimulation as indicated by the centre portion of the line.

What would the reaction be to this state of affairs of a cortex in a state of high excitation? We would expect on physiological grounds that a person of this type would experience all incoming stimulation more strongly than would the average person and consequently would be even more affected by strong painful stimulation, but would not object so much to sensory deprivation. Conversely, a person whose cortex was in a state of partial inhibition would be expected to tolerate pain rather better because some of the sensory input would be inhibited from reaching the cortex,[29] but he would all the more suffer from sensory deprivation. We can test this hypothesis quite easily by submitting known extraverts and introverts to conditions of painful stimulation and also to conditions of sensory deprivation.

When this was done it was found that indeed extraverts were very much more tolerant of pain but less tolerant of sensory deprivation than were introverts.

This general hypothesis may be summed up by saying that extraverts have a kind of 'stimulus hunger' which leads to some of the behaviour patterns we noted above. Thus their preference

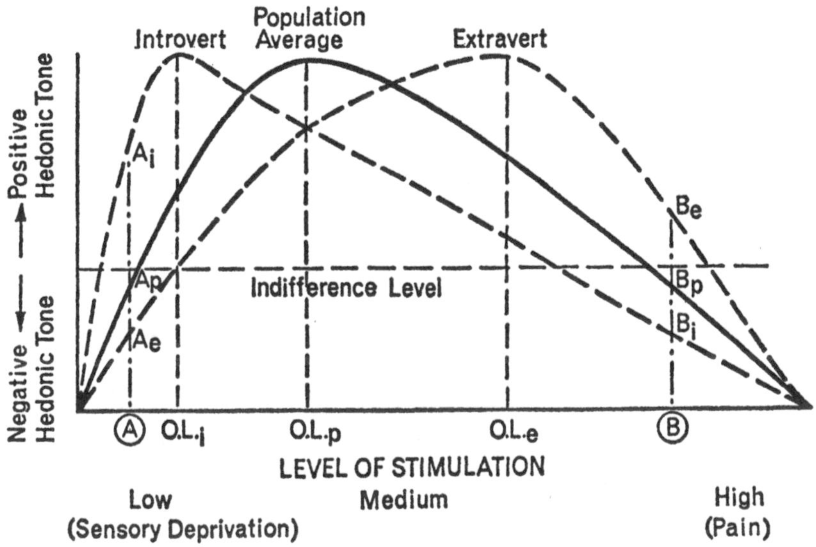

Fig. 21. Diagram showing relation between level of stimulation (abscissa) and hedonic tone (ordinate) in extraverts, introverts, and people not belonging to either extreme. Taken from H. J. Eysenck 'Experiments with Drugs', 1963. For explanation, see text.

for coffee and alcohol, for spicy foods, for premarital and extramarital intercourse, their impulsive and risk taking behaviour – all these can easily be deduced from this general hypothesis. We may similarly deduce from it that extraverts would be more likely to seek for the stimulation afforded by cigarette smoking, and it is on this basis that the original hypothesis was formulated. In addition we must consider the effects of nicotine itself. We have seen that nicotine is a stimulant drug thus having introverting effects. That means essentially that it produces a rise in the excitation of the cortex and thus in its efficiency. It counteracts inhibition and makes the person involved more likely to perceive, think, pay attention to and act more efficiently, particularly when he is otherwise in a state of lowered efficiency, such as might occur because of fatigue, illness or some other reason. As we posited a greater degree of inhibitory activity in the extravert he should be more in need of a stimulant drug and would therefore be more likely to seek one out. These are the two reasons then which lead us to predict that extraverts would be more likely to smoke cigarettes than would introverts.[30]

The writer has carried out two studies specifically to test this hypothesis. In the first of these a questionnaire was constructed which contained questions particularly relevant to extraversion and neuroticism.[31] Twenty-four groups of subjects were used, divided equally on the basis of age, (40–59 and 60–70), class (middle- and working-class), and smoking habits. There were 6 different groups classified according to smoking habit: non-smokers, light smokers, medium smokers, heavy smokers, pipe smokers and ex-smokers. There were approximately 100 subjects in each of the 24 groups. Random samples of the population were obtained for each of these groups, about 7,000 contacts being made by interviewers in order to locate the requisite number of subjects. A very careful sampling design was used in order to make sure that the population did in fact present us with a proper representative sample of the British Isles.

The results of the study are shown in Figure 22. It will be seen that the amount of extraversion increases as we go from non-smokers to light, to medium and finally to heavy smokers who are the most extraverted of all. Ex-smokers are situated between light and medium smokers as far as degree of extraversion is concerned; pipe smokers are the most introverted of all. The differences are fully significant statistically. This Figure and the results on which it is based thus strongly support our

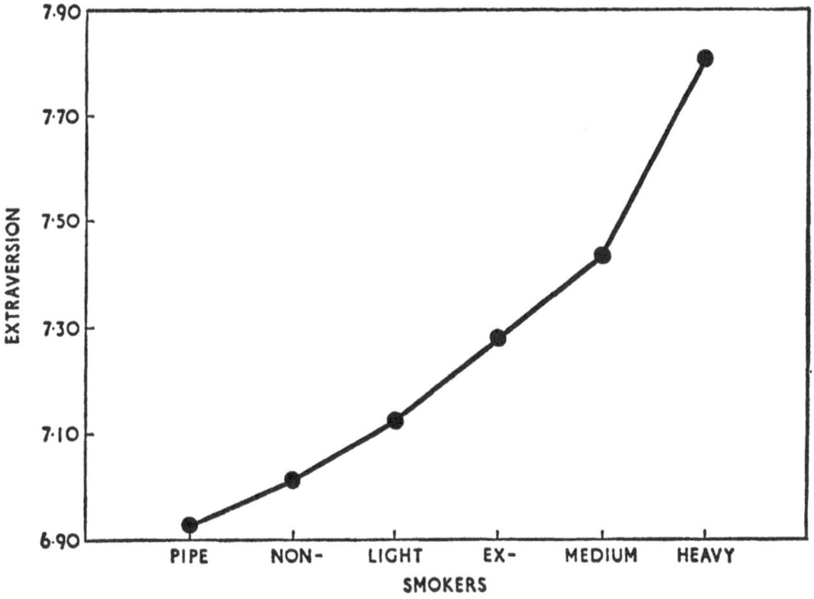

Fig. 22. Diagram showing relationship between scores on an extraversion questionnaire and smoking habits. There is an increase in cigarette smoking with increasing extraversion. Taken from H. J. Eysenck, *Life Sciences*, 1964, 3, 782. Data collected by Mass Observation.

hypothesis. It is interesting to note that in spite of the relatively large number of cases used there was no relationship between smoking and neuroticism.

A second inquiry was carried out to make certain that the results obtained were not statistical artefacts.[32] Again 24 subgroups were used as before containing roughly 100 male subjects all aged between 45 and 64 years. A rather different type of personality inventory was used; again neuroticism and extraversion were measured, but in addition care was taken to include separate measures of impulsiveness and sociability. Figure 23 shows the result of this study. Again it will be seen

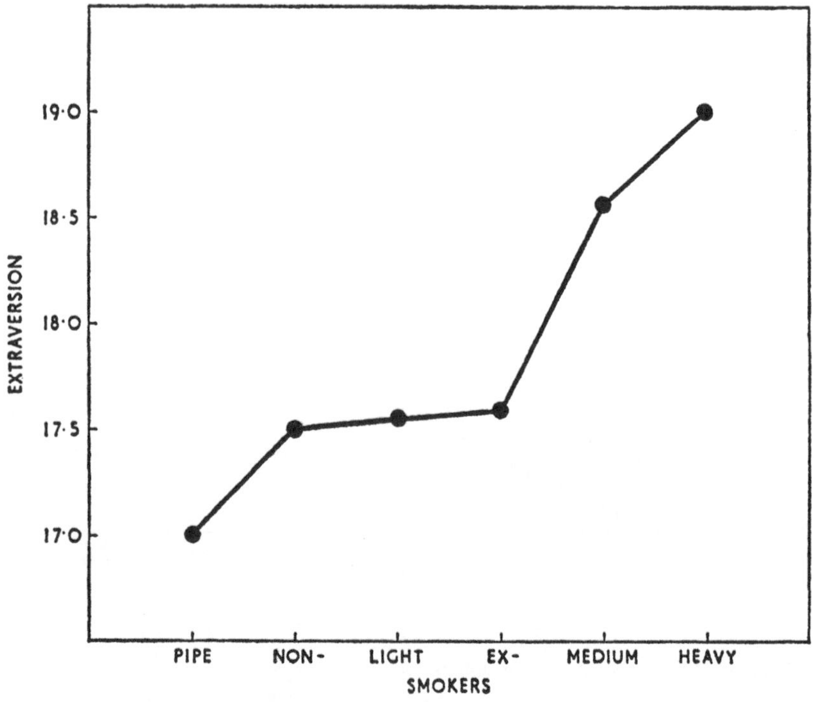

Fig. 23. Diagram showing results of another study linking extraversion and smoking habits and using a different questionnaire and population sample. Taken from H. J. Eysenck, *Life Sciences*, 1964, 3, 784. Data collected by Mass Observation.

that there is a regular progression in extraversion from non-smokers, through light, medium and to heavy smokers. Ex-smokers are between light and medium smokers and pipe smokers are again the most introverted group. Thus in every detail the main results of this study are similar to those of the first and support the hypothesis that the smoking of cigarettes is positively related to extraversion. Again it was found that no relationship existed between smoking and neuroticism. The separate scoring of traits of sociability and impulsiveness did not add any information, as these traits were not related to smoking apart from the contribution they made to the measurement of extraversion.

Are these findings supported by results obtained by other workers? The answer on the whole must be yes. Consider the following findings.[33] It has been shown that cigarette smokers also tend to partake more frequently of coffee and of alcoholic beverages; we have already noted before that extraverts tend to drink more coffee and more liquor. Cigarette smokers are known to be more frequently involved in driving accidents; it has been found that extraverts tend to be more frequently involved in driving accidents than are introverts. It has been found that divorced people tend to smoke more whereas single people tend not to smoke; we have already noted that introverts tend to marry less and extraverts to be more frequently involved in a change of marital partner. It has been found that people who change jobs frequently tend to smoke more; again extraverts are known to change jobs more frequently. Several studies have tended to show that people who are relatively unsuccessful academically, both at school and university, tend to smoke more; it has also been found that introverts are more successful at school and at university. People who smoke a lot have been found to be 'chance oriented'; this agrees well with the findings that extraverts tend to be impulsive. Last it has been found that on various personality questionnaires of gregariousness, social introversion, and the Pd scale of the M.M.P.I. smokers score in the extraverted direction. All these findings come from American studies and they all support the generalization that cigarette smoking is correlated with extraversion.

Many American studies have also been concerned with neuroticism or emotionality, and it must be said that here agreement is much less obvious. Most of the American studies have found a positive relationship between smoking and neuroticism. Admittedly many of these studies were carried out on relatively small groups, and in most cases groups chosen were quite unrepresentative. Nevertheless, the amount of agreement reported must make one cautious of dismissing these results. The American report summarizes the findings in the following sentence: 'Despite the individual deficiencies of many of the studies, despite the great diversity in conceptualization and research methods used and despite discrepancies in reported findings the presence of some comparability between them and the relative consistency of findings lend support to the existence of a relationship between the smoking habit and a personality configuration that is vaguely described as "neurotic".' The tortured structure and syntax of this sentence adequately indicate the difficulty which the authors had in coming to a conclusion on this point; it must be left to further research to say whether the difference between our findings and those mentioned are due to national differences between England and America or whether there is some other cause for the discrepancy.

There is one further set of data which may be mentioned in this connection. Body build is almost certainly determined by constitutional factors, and it has been shown many times that there is a relationship between extraversion/introversion and body build.[34] It is customary to define body build in terms of a continuum, one extreme of which shows a long lean type of body whereas the other shows a squat, thick-set type of physique. The former is often called 'leptosomatic', the other 'pyknic' or 'athletic'. (Sometimes the thick-set type of physique is subdivided again into two, the fat (pyknic) and the muscular (athletic).) The evidence shows that introverts tend to be leptosomatic in body build, while extraverts tend to be pyknic or athletic. If our hypothesis linking extraversion to smoking is correct then we should expect that smokers would be pyknic or athletic in body build. Is this true?

R. W. Parnell carried out a study in Oxford in 1951 on 308 undergraduates. He found that students of leptosomatic body build were the least frequent smokers, whereas the most frequent ones were pyknics, with athletic body build students somewhere in the middle. C. B. Thomas studied more than 1,000 students at the Johns Hopkins University School of Medicine in Baltimore. She found that there was an excess of smokers who were 30 per cent or more overweight and that subjects who were 40 per cent or more overweight were more regular smokers. The non-smokers had a greater frequency of individuals with 10 per cent or more underweight than the smokers. C. C. Seltzer followed up a group of almost 1,000 Harvard students over a period of thirteen years and found that the smokers had larger dimensions than the non-smokers, being greater than non-smokers in height, weight, in the dimensions of the head, face, shoulders, chest, hip, leg and hand. All these studies are in agreement with our hypothesis showing that smokers tend to be more pyknic in body build and also usually more athletic than are non-smokers, who tend to be leptosomatic.

There is one study carried out by A. Damon which appears to go counter to this trend. However, he was concerned with a very small sample of very unusual composition, dealing with 167 adult male factory workers of Neapolitan parentage but of American birth and upbringing. He found that lean men tended to smoke more than stout or fat (but not muscular) men, but such a finding must be viewed against a background of the curious racial and national composition of his small sample, and it is doubtful whether it can be used to throw doubt on the concordant findings of all the other studies which used much larger and more homogeneous groups of subjects.[35]

Our general conclusion then from studies of personality, social behaviour and body build is that cigarette smokers on the whole tend to show extraverted behaviour patterns and that this relationship is a quantitative one, i.e. the greater the number of cigarettes smoked the greater is the degree of extraversion of the smokers concerned. It is unfortunate that no information is available on the manner of smoking; it is quite likely that extraverts do not only smoke more cigarettes but also smoke them more greedily, i.e. take more puffs, take stronger puffs and smoke their cigarettes down to a shorter butt. There are no differences between extraverts and introverts with respect to inhaling but it is interesting to note that such differences do exist with respect to neuroticism. The more neurotic tend to inhale more regardless of whether they are light smokers, medium smokers or heavy smokers. Even ex-smokers when asked to report on their past habits show a difference with respect to this personality trait. Until further studies have been carried out, however, nothing more can be said about any possible differences between extraverts and introverts, or the stable and unstable, as regards their mode of smoking.

Chapter 6

Cancer and Personality

For thy sake, Tobacco, I
Would do any thing but die.
CHARLES LAMB

THE NOTION THAT constitutional factors play an important part in the causation of diseases is a very ancient one. Hippocrates, who lived in the fifth century BC, described the two main types of body build we have already referred to and suggested that the pyknic type is predisposed to develop apoplexy whereas the leptosomatic type was predisposed to develop tuberculosis. Galen whom we have also already encountered suggested that cancer was more much frequent in 'melancholic' than in 'sanguine' women; thus relating disease not only to constitution but directly to personality. This notion was very much in the air during the nineteenth century, and in 1802 a group of leading physicians in England formed 'The Society for the Prevention and Cure of Cancer'. They suggested a variety of points on which they felt there was a need for further research; one of these was 'Is there a predisposing temperament?' Much clinical research was done during the subsequent years and in 1846 W. H. Walshe, in his book *Nature and Treatment of Cancer* claimed that there seemed to be general agreement that 'women of high colour and sanguinous temperament were more subject to mammary cancer than those of different constitution.'

All this may come as a surprise to many people who believe that the notion of psychosomatic diseases is a fairly recent one and owes its inception to Freud and other psychoanalytic writers. Quite the opposite is true. During the nineteenth century the hypothesis of psychosomatic disorders was not only generally accepted by most medical people but it was extended to diseases which even today most psychiatrists would believe to be outside this general field.[36] It was only towards the end of the nineteenth century that the whole idea fell into disfavour. This disfavour, it may be added in parentheses, was well deserved. Very far-reaching claims were made with very little basis in fact; experimental methods of inquiry were eschewed; and there was usually little agreement between different workers. Even in the little that we have quoted the reader will already have noted very clear evidence of disagreement. Thus according to Galen cancer was much more frequent in melancholic women; according to Walshe, however, it was much more frequent in sanguine women. Whom are we to believe?

It is notable that the resurgence of the hypothesis of psychosomatic disease, i.e. of the interaction between psychological factors and disease-producing processes, which has taken place in recent years, has not improved to any very great extent on this state of affairs. Much of the so-called research is still of an anecdotal nature. There is little experimental evidence one way or the other, and different investigators show the same tendency to contradict each other's findings as was true during the last century. For these reasons many medical people refuse to take seriously the very idea of psychosomatic diseases and critics usually add that the very notion of psychological factors influencing disease processes is not one that recommends itself to the scientific temperament.

In principle the writer would agree with this criticism if by personality we understand some mystical principle superimposed upon physiological and neurological processes and entirely separate from them. The Cartesian separation of body and mind has been responsible in the past for idealistic views of personality of this kind. However, it will be noted that the type of theory which we have put forward in this book is not subject to criticisms of this nature. As has been pointed out, the main dimensions of personality are determined by inherited structures of the central and autonomic nervous systems, and it does not take a very great act of faith to imagine that inherited differences in these structures may also aid or inhibit the inception and spreading of a variety of diseases. Nicotine, for instance, is known to stimulate the autonomic nervous system, and we have also already noted that the autonomic system is very closely linked with the expression of the emotions and with the factor of neuroticism. It thus constitutes a mediating link between any possible effect that nicotine may have on health and temperament on the other hand. To say this, of course, does not by itself get us very far; clearly what is necessary is a very detailed and experimental working out of the relations involved. What may be claimed, however, is that the idea of psychosomatic interaction is not one which is necessarily remote from scientific understanding.

One hypothesis which was widely held during the nineteenth century was that psychological shock might be in part responsible for the development of cancers. Walshe, whom we have already quoted, put the case extremely well when he wrote: 'Much has been written on the influence of mental misery, sudden reverses of fortune, and habitual gloominess of temper on the deposition of carcinomatous matter. If systematic writers can be credited these constitute the most powerful cause of the disease . . . although the alleged influence of mental disquietude has never been made a matter of demonstration it will be vain to deny that facts of a very convincing character in respect to the agency of the mind and the production of this disease are frequently observed. I have myself met with cases in which the connection appeared so clear that I decided questioning its reality would have seemed a struggle against reason.' Some more experimental work has been recently done in this connection and the results on the whole seem to support this idea.[37] When cancer patients and non-cancer patients are compared it is more frequently among the former than the latter that some recent event has occurred causing psychological shock to the patient. However, the literature is by no means unanimous and the methods of investigation used have not been of a kind to recommend themselves to experimentalists. Nevertheless, it would be premature to dismiss the idea as wholly absurd; some much more satisfactory recent work by D. M. Kissen in connection with tuberculosis, where a similar view has long been held, has produced evidence which is much more acceptable and which seems to support this view.[38]

Is there any more direct and acceptable evidence linking cancer with constitutional factors and with the personality factors we have considered so far? We have shown that there is a tendency for extraverts to smoke cigarettes more and we have also found that extraverts tend to have a body build which is distinctive, i.e. they tend to be pyknic or athletic. If our hypothesis of a constitutional factor underlying both cancer and smoking be correct then we would expect persons suffering from cancer to have a pyknic or athletic type of body build rather than a leptosomatic one. Some light is thrown on this point by data collected by the American psychologist, W. H. Sheldon, who has made a special investigation of the body build of varieties of patients, some suffering from tuberculosis, others from cancer of the breast and cancer of the uterus. Also included among his groups were American students and American delinquents. Figure 24 shows the outcome of a comparison of these various groups. It will be seen that the patients suffering from tuberculosis tend to be the most leptosomatic, delinquents seem to be fairly pyknic and athletic, and the cancer patients, whether suffering from cancer of the breast or cancer of the uterus, are the most pyknic/athletic of the lot. The data are really quite surprising in their definite separation of the cancer patients from the tuberculosis patients: almost half of the tuberculosis patients are more leptosomatic than the most leptosomatic of all the cancer patients! It would be easy to make too much of these findings, particularly as the two cancer groups were not specifically concerned with cancer of the lung, but

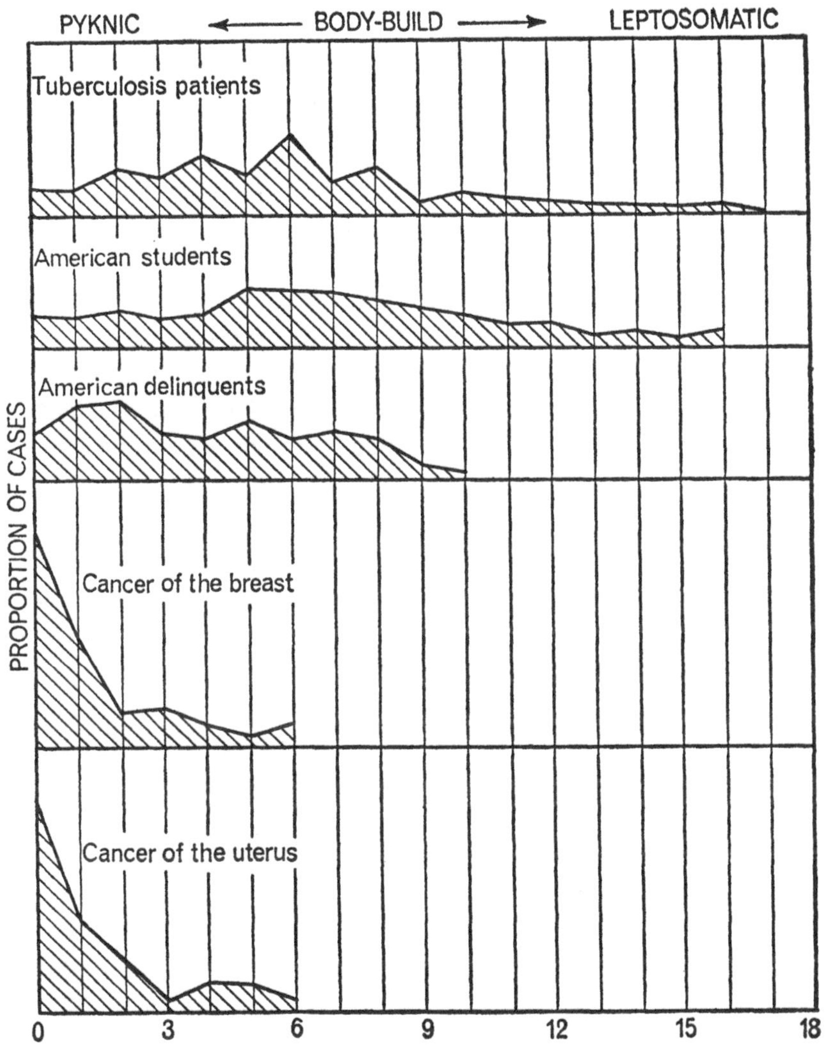

Fig. 24. Relationship between body build and various diseases. It will be seen that sufferers from tuberculosis tend to be leptosomatic (lean), whereas cancer patients tend to be stocky in body build. Delinquents tend to be somewhat stocky, students somewhat lean. The figure is quoted from H. J. Eysenck 'Fact and Fiction in Psychology', 1965; the data are taken from W. H. Sheldon, *et al.*, 'Varieties of Delinquent Youths', 1949.

nevertheless the agreement with hypothesis cannot be overlooked.

Studies of body build are one thing; studies of personality are another. The first to link personality with cancer was a Swedish doctor, O. Hagnell, who reported on the results of an epidemiological survey of the 2,550 inhabitants of two adjacent rural parishes in the south of Sweden.[39] This survey was started in 1947 and included an interview during which a personality assessment was made on each subject. Ten years later the procedure was repeated and the subsequent history of each subject examined. During this follow-up it was observed that a significantly high proportion of women who had developed cancer had been originally rated as extraverted. Actually, Hagnell used a rather different system of personality assessment to the one used here, but there is considerable evidence that the particular set of qualities which he found associated with cancer was in fact similar to or identical with what we have called extraversion. Hagnell also noted relationships between cancer and body build.

The next study to appear in the literature was carried out by D. M. Kissen and the present writer; it appeared in 1962.[40] The Maudsley Personality Inventory (M.P.I.), designed by the present author, was used to measure the two personality dimensions of extraversion and neuroticism. The persons studied consisted of patients admitted to three chest units for diagnosis and treatment. Two of these units were surgical units and contained not only patients in whom lung cancer might be expected but also patients admitted with other suspected thoracic disorders. Patients from a medical chest unit were also included. Patients were interviewed by Dr Kissen and in no case was the diagnosis known to the interviewer at the time of the interview. Altogether 239 patients were seen, in 116 of whom a diagnosis of primary lung cancer was made, and in 123 of whom cancer of any organ was excluded. There was no refusals and all the patients were males. A special aspect of the study was the division of each group into two, depending on whether they had or had not previously suffered from psychosomatic disorders. Furthermore, the patients were subdivided into groups according to age, the first group with ages below 55, the second with ages from 55 to 64, and the third with ages of 65 upwards.

Taking extraversion first it was found that there were hardly any differences between cancer and control patients when the groups without psychosomatic disorder were compared. In comparing the groups with psychosomatic disorder however it was found that the cancer group was considerably more extraverted than the control group. Higher extraversion scores of the cancer patients were found in all three age groups but most strongly in the middle one (55–64 years). The results are not particularly striking and it is not quite clear why patients with and without psychosomatic disorders should differ in respect to the relationship that cancer shows to extraversion. Nevertheless, as far as they go they are roughly in conformity with expectation; extraverts on the whole tend to be more likely to be suffering from lung cancer.

When we look at the neuroticism scores it is surprising to note that the control group has much higher scores than the cancer group regardless of psychosomatic involvement. The data are fully significant statistically and the differences are quite surprisingly high. These results were interpreted by D. M. Kissen as supporting a theory he had formulated on the basis of a long series of psycho-social studies on lung cancer patients. During the course of these studies, he writes, 'some of the clinical material elicited suggested the hypothesis that lung cancer patients had a significantly diminished outlet for emotional discharge compared with non-cancer patients'. The present study he felt supported this view quite strongly.

The next study to report on the relationship between cancer and extraversion was carried out by Dr Alec Coppen and Mrs Maryse Metcalfe of the Medical Research Council Neuropsychiatric Research Unit. [41] They also used the M.P.I. for their inquiry.[42] Working in a general hospital they used patients in two gynaecological and two surgical wards, and outpatients attending the surgical clinic. Questionnaires were first filled in by the patients, and at the end of the investigations the questionnaires were collected and scored and the diagnosis of each patient obtained. Forty-seven patients had a malignant tumour, 32 had cancer of the breast, 4 had cancer of the uterus and 11 had cancer in other parts of the body. Two control groups were used; one was a hospital control group made up of 129 patients with various gynaecological and surgical conditions. Care was taken that these should all fall into the same age group as the patients with cancer. A second control group of 31 subjects was obtained from a representative sample of the general population of the London area. This control group was somewhat younger than the hospital groups and therefore these subjects would be expected to have had higher extraversion scores than the cancer group on account of their age alone. The mean extraversion scores of the hospital controls and the general population controls were very similar. The cancer group, however, had significantly higher extraversion scores than both control groups. Their mean neuroticism scores did not differ significantly. The sub-groups of cancer patients had all very similar means.

Coppen and Metcalfe go on to discuss certain hormonal differences related to body build and personality; they conclude that 'although the nature of this association is by no means clear one may perhaps speculate that certain constitutional factors predispose individuals to develop malignant tumours. Extraversion may be one manifestation of this constitutional difference which may also be related to physique and to hormonal activity.' This study, too, then finds a relationship between cancer (although primarily not cancer of the lung) and extraversion; no correlation is found with neuroticism.

The last study to be discussed was carried out by D. M. Kissen who further pursued the theory of a relationship between lung cancer and lack of neuroticism which we have already noted.[43] In this study, which was published in 1964, he reports on the neuroticism scores on the M.P.I. of lung cancer patients and other chest unit admissions. Again it is found that the lung cancer patients are very significantly lower on neuroticism scores than are the other patients. Kissen gives a rather interesting table in which he calculates lung cancer mortality rates per 100,000 men aged 25 and over by levels of neuroticism scores. He finds that people with very low scores have a mortality rate of 296, those with intermediate scores have a mortality rate of 108 and those with very high scores have a mortality rate of only 56. He assumes, of course, that men aged 25 and over suffering respectively from lung cancer and non-chest diseases can be taken as representing male lung cancer deaths and men generally in Scotland, an assumption which is almost certainly not an accurate representation of the facts but which is perhaps not too far removed from the actual state of affairs to pass muster. He must also assume, of course, that samples of 100 each are large enough to make meaningful comparisons possible; clearly there is a wide margin here for considerable chance effects. Nevertheless, the figures are statistically significant and as they are quoted present quite amazingly great differences between people having high and low scores respectively on the neuroticism scale of the M.P.I. When it is realized that these are raw figures, i.e. uncorrected for attenuation due to lack of perfect reliability and validity of the scales it will be realized that there is considerable support here for the assumption of a relationship between the development of lung cancer and constitutional personality factors.

It would not be feasible to interpret these data as necessarily supporting Dr Kissen's hypothesis. He assumes that low scores on a neuroticism questionnaire can be used as indicative of poor outlets for emotional discharge in persons giving such scores. An alternative hypothesis of course might be that these people simply do not have very strong emotions to discharge, and this interpretation is very much more in line with the information we have on people scoring high and low on this questionnaire. However, interpretation of facts is one thing and the provision of facts is another, and there can be no doubt that Dr Kissen has been successful in producing facts which will require much thought and much further work before their import can be properly digested.

Before summarizing our results it is interesting to note that some studies have also been carried out on the relationship between personality and coronary artery disease. Dr Wilde compared 34 male outpatients with myocardial infarction with a population sample of 1,887 and found that the patients were characterized by a more than average degree of neuroticism and a more than average degree of extraversion; in other words they fell into the 'choleric' quadrant of our Figure.[44] Some unpublished American studies have also given results implicating extraversion in coronary disease. All this, of course, is not directly relevant to the problem of lung cancer, but it will be remembered that coronary disease was statistically related to smoking almost as strongly as lung cancer and it is certainly interesting to find that both diseases are significantly related to a common personality trait, namely extraversion. They differ, of course, with respect to neuroticism or emotionality, lung cancer patients being less emotional than the average person whereas sufferers from coronary artery disease are more emotional.

How can we summarize the data reported in this brief chapter? In the first place note that the chapter is indeed very brief and that the number of investigations quoted is very small. The reason for this unfortunate state of affairs is, of course, that very few people have shown any interest in the notion of constitutional factors in disease generally and in cancer specifically. The present climate of medical opinion stresses very much the nature and discovery of the disease-producing agent and does not concern itself to anything like the same extent with the infected organism. While this is the general atmosphere in which research is conducted it is unlikely that we will discover much of a change in the disproportion of effort which is devoted to these two different sides of the medal.

The second point which emerges is that the evidence on the

whole tends to support the view that constitutional factors in general and personality factors in particular are correlated with proneness to cancer. The evidence is stronger in relation to cancer as such than it is in relation to lung cancer alone. But even there the results are positive and quite suggestive. On the whole it would appear that people suffering from lung cancer tend to be extraverted, particularly when they are also suffering from psychosomatic disorders, and to be rather low on neuroticism. In other words, they seem to fall into the 'sanguine' part of our Figure 16, and it is curious to remember that Walshe, writing over one hundred years ago, had already suggested such a relationship. Perhaps the medical old wives' tales that we mentioned at the beginning of this chapter may have had some more truth in them than was recognized at the time or even later!

Our third conclusion from the data examined must be that interesting though the results are, and promising as this approach appears, yet nevertheless it would be unscientific to claim too much for what has been established. The results are suggestive, they are congruent with each other, and they fit in with the general theoretical framework developed on previous pages. Nevertheless, the numbers involved are relatively small and there are many unanswered questions remaining, such as for instance the interaction between the personality/cancer association and psychosomatic disorders. Clearly the situation cannot be left where it is. What is required is a much greater involvement of research activity in this field, the use of much larger numbers of subjects, and possibly even the subdivision of lung cancer patients into the various types of lung cancer we have described on a previous page. Furthermore, while questionnaires are useful devices in giving a rough and ready picture of personality, they are far from being perfect instruments of measurement as far as constitutional factors are concerned; it can be calculated that the *true* relationships between a given variable and personality are likely to be something like four times as strong as those discovered by the use of questionnaires.

The loss of 75 per cent of the association is due to attenuation connected with lack of reliability and lack of validity of the measuring instrument. Such losses are, of course, very serious, and it is surprising that the data we have discussed are as positive as they are in view of this loss. This means, however, that for future work more experimental types of test are likely to prove of value, and these can only be administered in properly equipped laboratories, air-conditioned and sound-proofed. These, unfortunately, are seldom found in hospitals dealing with patients of the kind we wish to investigate.

In conclusion it may be useful to discuss briefly one further point which may have occurred to the reader. Is it not possible, he may ask, that the relationship between disease and extraversion have been mediated through the agency of cigarette smoking? In other words, is it not possible that extraverts develop lung cancer and other types of cancer more readily simply because they smoke more than do introverts? Most of the studies mentioned have been on the outlook for this effect, and the answer must be in the negative. A very small proportion of the relationship may possibly be due to this factor, but it cannot by any stretch of the imagination be held responsible for the total effect. This is even more true, of course, of the relationship between lung cancer and neuroticism where in any case no mediating factor can be postulated due to the absence of any relationship between neuroticism and smoking (if any such relationship were to be discovered it would most likely be in the opposite direction in any case, i.e. people with high scores on neuroticism smoke more, people with low scores on neuroticism develop lung cancer!).

Chapter 7

The Causes of Lung Cancer

Youk'n hide de fier, but w'at you gwine do wid de smoke?
JOEL CHANDLER HARRIS

IT WILL HAVE become clear to the reader that even if cigarette smoking is responsible for lung cancer to some extent, it is neither a *necessary* nor a *sufficient* cause for that or any other disease. Ten per cent of lung cancer cases occur among non-smokers; this proves that smoking is not necessary in order to have people die from lung cancer. Similarly, it has been found that one in every eleven men aged 25 who smoked more than 25 cigarettes a day will die of lung cancer before attaining the age of 75; that means that 10 out of 11 who smoked this quite large number of cigarettes would survive without lung cancer. For those smoking between 15 and 25 cigarettes a day 1 man in 20 died of lung cancer; this leaves 19 out of 20 smoking moderately who would not at any time contract lung cancer. Thus cigarette smoking is not a sufficient cause of lung cancer either; the majority of those who smoke even in excess are not liable to die of the disease. These undisputed facts are seldom stated in quite this way, but I think it useful and valuable to be clear on this point.

It is precisely because smoking at most is neither a necessary nor a sufficient cause that it is so difficult to prove that is is a cause at all. In using the term 'cause' here we have, of course, to fall foul of modern philosophical discussions which have brought the whole concept of causation into some disrepute. The term is being used entirely in its common sense meaning and it would be quite an unnecessary exercise to try and rephrase perfectly clear-cut sentences in order to accommodate philosophical refinement. However, certain consequences follow from this general statement about smoking as a cause of cancer, and it will be the task of this chapter to investigate some of these.

When we say that smoking is not a necessary cause of cancer we are saying in effect that there are a number of other causes and it becomes important to find out just what these are. One of the best attested is simply urbanization, i.e. the factor of more and more people living in greater proximity to each other. Figure 25 shows the male lung cancer standardized mortality ratios for lung cancer in urban and rural districts in England over the period 1952 to 1960. It will be seen that the ratios are very much higher for the urban than for the rural populations, and it is important to note that these differences are not themselves due to smoking.[45] The relation between lung cancer rates and degrees of urbanization is in fact a linear one. In other words, the greater the degree of urbanization the greater the death rate from lung cancer. This is shown in Figure 26 which gives rate of lung cancer in men per 100,000 for six different types of living areas in England beginning with London and passing through conurbations, county boroughs, other urban districts, total rural districts to truly rural districts in order of smaller and smaller number of persons per acre. It will be seen that there is a corresponding fall in the lung cancer death rate, with London having a death rate in 1951 about four times as high as truly rural districts. Urbanization, therefore, appears to be a very powerful factor in lung cancer.

Now clearly the concept of 'urbanization' cannot be used in any sensible way to denote a causal factor by itself; it must be something more specific connected with urbanization which is responsible. There is evidence from the animal field that simply increasing the number of animals in a given area beyond a certain point causes deterioration in behaviour and health; these experiments are sometimes known by the title of 'behaviour sink' to denote this general incapacity to adapt to overcrowding.

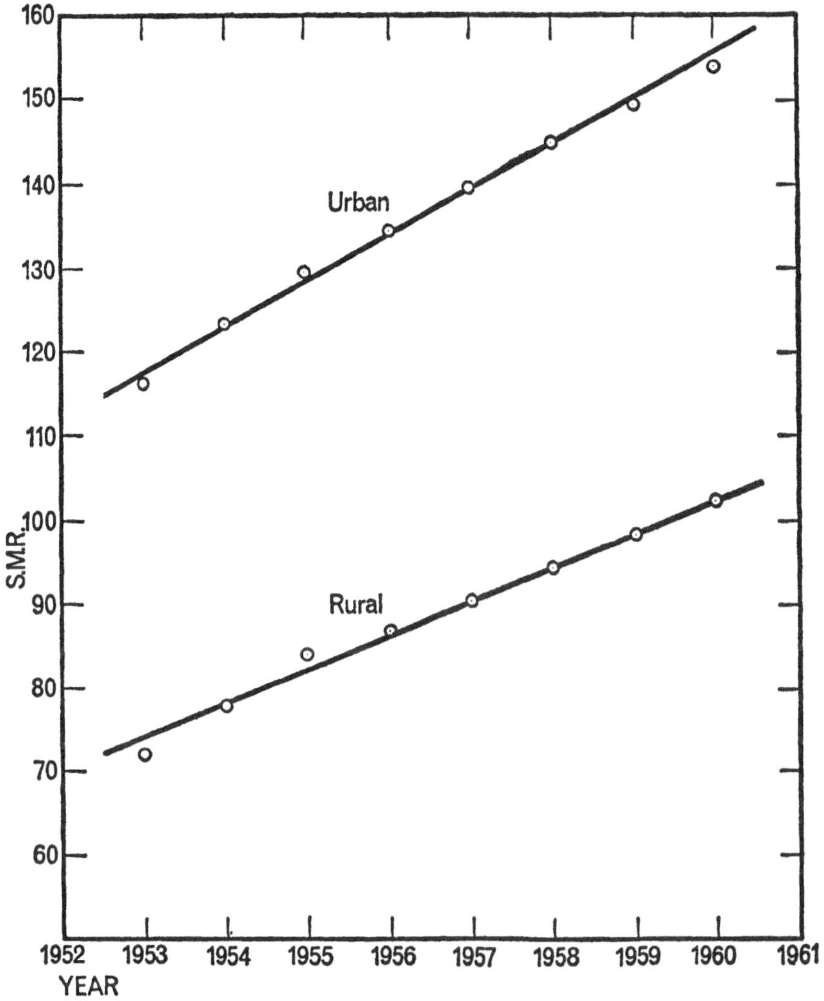

Fig. 25. Incidence and increase of standardized mortality rates for male lung cancer in urban and rural districts in England. Taken with permission from S. F. Buck and D. A. Brown, *Tobacco Research Council Research Papers, No. 7*, 28.

That overcrowding can indeed affect not only behaviour but the actual physical processes underlying disease and protection therefrom is shown by many animal experiments in which it

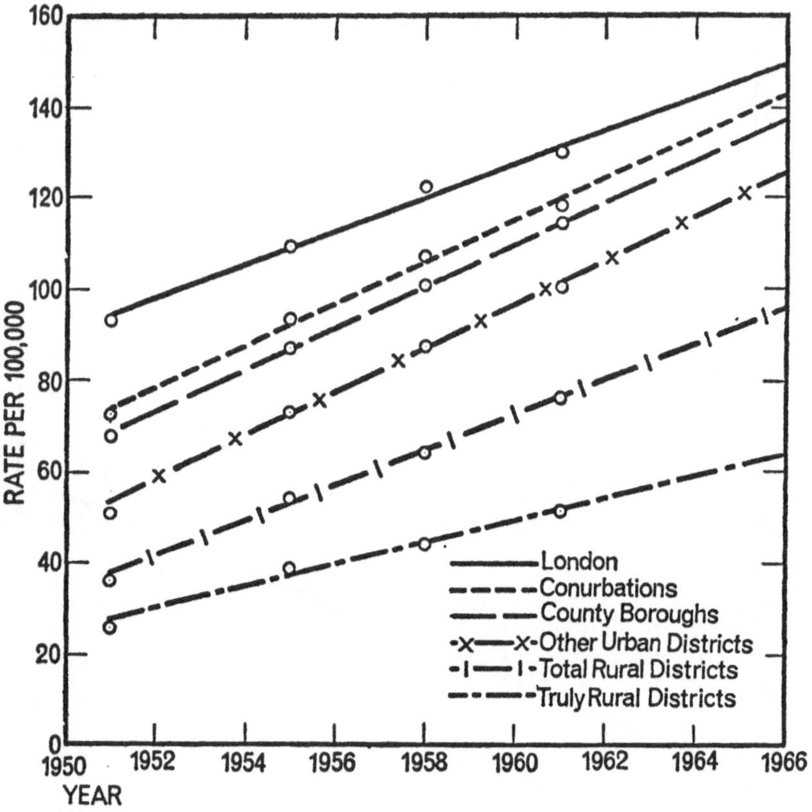

Fig. 26. Urban /rural variations in lung cancer in England and Wales for men. Taken with permission from S. F. Buck and D. A. Brown, *Tobacco Research Council Research Papers, No. 7*, 29.

has been found that the lethal dose of various drugs is much lower for animals living in crowded conditions than for animals living alone. Recently, S. Vesey and D. E. Davis have reported on experiments in which they kept some mice in groups of 6 while others were kept in isolation. All the animals received injections of beef serum, a foreign protein which stimulates the production of antibodies. They discovered that the lonely mice produced significantly higher concentrations of antibodies than did those living in crowded conditions, thus receiving greater protection. In another experiment Vesey and Davis gave the mice tetanus toxin injections, a highly poisonous substance produced by tetanus bacilli against which the body usually protects itself by producing antibodies. Of 40 mice so injected and living in groups, 33 died; out of 30 mice living alone only 11 died. These results are typical of many others, and the whole problem is considered in some detail by Richard Fiennes in his book *Man, Nature and Disease*, in which he suggests that wild animals usually live in a state of balance in which infectious diseases are not of great importance. Overcrowding, however, may lead to a breakdown of this equilibrium and thus to disease.

The study by Buck and Brown referred to above does indeed lead to the conclusion that the association with lung cancer mortality is primarily due to population density, and this is a clue which ought certainly to be followed up in future work. In terms of our biological inheritance, living overcrowded lives in gigantic cities is certainly 'unnatural' and may have deleterious effects. It is difficult to see, however, why these effects should manifest themselves particularly in relation to lung cancer and only if more definitive and detailed evidence is forthcoming will this particular aspect of 'urbanization' need to be taken seriously.

Much more impressive is the evidence relating to air pollution. The case here has been argued particularly strongly by Pybus whose account we will follow.[46] He points out to begin with that the first important discovery regarding the causes of cancer was made by a London surgeon, Percival Pott, who, in 1775, described cancer of the scrotum in chimney sweeps and decided it was due to soot lodged in the crevices of the skin of the male genitals. 'This cancer occurred almost entirely in adults, but not by any means in all sweeps, and only after many years' contamination. . . . One of the peculiarities of cancer is often the long latent period which may elapse before the disease shows itself. . . . Another important fact emerged in 1892 when a London surgeon, H. D. Butlin, again studied Chimney Sweep's cancer and wondered about its occurrence among continental sweeps. He inquired of a number of surgeons in the main European cities, who replied that while they knew of its existence amongst British sweeps, they had never seen a case. Surprised at this information, Butlin and his assistants visited these cities and found that the continental sweeps were cleanly and prevented the soot reaching or remaining in contact with their skin, in contrast to the British sweeps, whose bodies, clothing and houses were soot-ridden; hence the deduction, "No soot, no cancer".'

The apparent causal relationship between soot, the tar contained in it and the production of skin cancer led to a series of experiments with animals in which tar was painted on their skins; success was finally achieved in 1915 when a skin cancer was produced on a rabbit by tar painting. In 1925 it was shown that tar (condensed smoke) from burning a variety of materials would cause cancer if applied to the skin in sufficient quantity.

'It seemed obvious that in the tar, soot and mineral oil there must be one or more substances capable of converting the normal cells of the skin into those whose behaviour should be such as to constitute cancer. That is, the cell, previously well behaved, and performing its normal useful functions, was so altered that it multiplied far beyond the body's needs, invaded the surrounding parts, replaced some tissues, was carried to distant organs which it destroyed, and almost invariably caused death.

'In 1930, after many years of investigation, Kennaway and others succeeded not only in detecting and isolating one important cancer-producing chemical, benzpyrene, but also in making it. Since 1930, a host of substances have proved to be mildly or strongly carcinogenic though benzpyrene is the most important and is found almost universally in SMOKE. Benzpyrene also occurs in tar, soot and other coal tar products so that we have the explanation why these substances have been causing cancer of the skin over the centuries. Both benzpyrene and the other carcinogenic substances which may be found in smoke are cyclic hydrocarbons.'

We thus have now a logical indictment of smoke as a possible cause of cancer and it is interesting to note two facts. The first is that coal consumption in Great Britain as in most other countries has been rising until quite recently so that the curve of its consumption closely parallels the growth of lung cancer. The second fact is brought out clearly in Table 2, which is quoted from Pybus. This shows that the total amount of benzpyrene produced by coal smoke per year in Great Britain is 750 tons, that produced by tobacco smoke is 8 lbs! Even allowing for the fact that tobacco smoke is probably brought into more intimate contact with the lungs the difference is suggestive, and it should be noted that the comparison does not include other sources of atmospheric pollution such as petroleum products which also contain benzpyrene, and smoke produced by the burning of vegetable matter as in bonfires, etc.

TABLE 2

COMPARISON OF ATMOSPHERIC POLLUTION
(per year in Great Britain)

COAL SMOKE	TOBACCO SMOKE
Coal burnt: *180 million tons*	Tobacco burnt: *111,607 tons*
Smoke formed: *2·5 million tons*	Smoke formed: *18,000 tons*
Concentration of benzpyrene in coal smoke: *300 parts per million*	Concentration of benzpyrene in tobacco smoke: *0·2 parts per million*
Total benzpyrene: *750 tons*	Total benzpyrene: *8 pounds*

Taken with permission from F. C. Pybus, *Newcastle Med. J.*, 1963, **28**, 42.

The figures regarding total benzpyrene production due to coal smoke are probably in excess of the true figures; Professor Pybus in a private communication has informed me that only half of the coal used is smoke producing and that therefore the figure for the total benzpyrene may be as low as 400 tons or thereabouts. This does not of course alter the general conclusion to be drawn from this table.

Some interesting and more direct evidence for the relation between smoke and hydrocarbons in the air comes from the work of Stocks and is shown in Figure 27 which gives the amount of smoke in twenty-six cities as related to the amount of hydrocarbons in the air.[47] Stocks has also given information about the relationship between lung cancer and amount of smoke in the air and this is shown in Figure 28; it will be seen that in

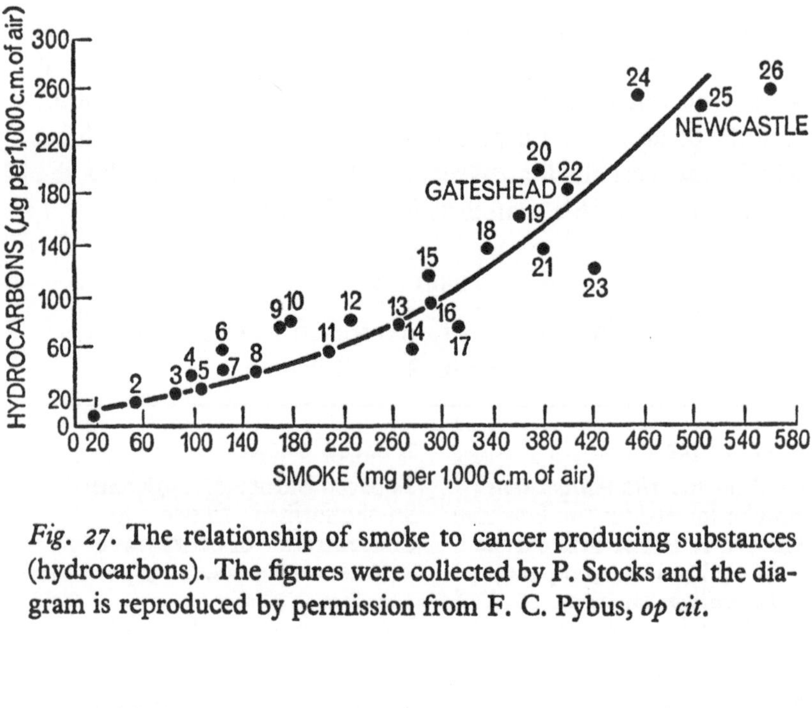

Fig. 27. The relationship of smoke to cancer producing substances (hydrocarbons). The figures were collected by P. Stocks and the diagram is reproduced by permission from F. C. Pybus, *op cit.*

areas with the least amount of smoke the incidence of lung cancer is only a quarter of what it is in areas with the greatest amount of smoke. Stocks also investigated the relationship between smoke and other types of cancer; this relationship is very much less clear cut than that with lung cancer, as one might have expected. The evidence implicating air pollution, therefore, seems to be very strong, although it must be stated that some investigators have failed to find as strong a relation between smoke and lung cancer as did Stocks in his original studies.[48] Here too, clearly, much further work is required to bring out the precise facts in the situation.

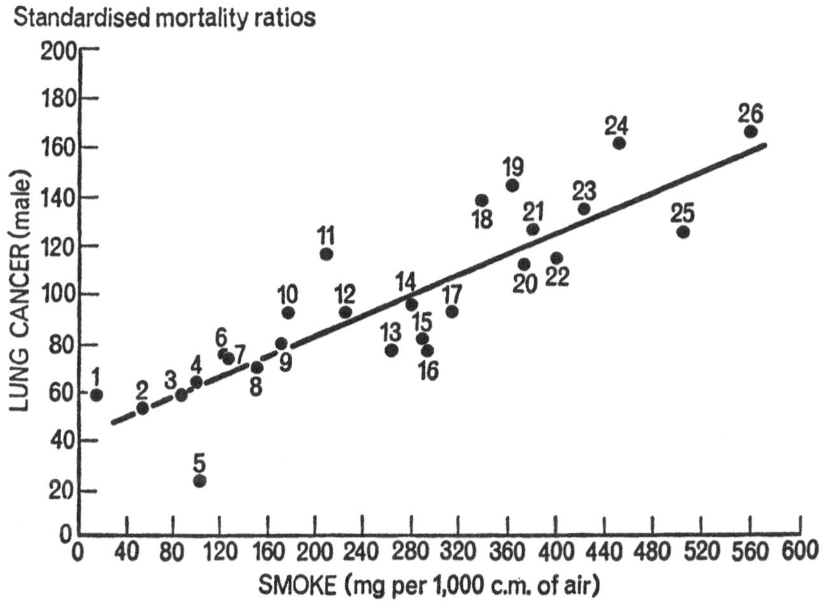

Fig. 28. Lung cancer rate in males in 26 different locations, differing widely in amount of smoke in the atmosphere. The figures were collected by P. Stocks and the diagram is reproduced by permission from F. C. Pybus, *op cit.*

There is, however, another interesting line of evidence produced by Eastcott. He found that the death rate from lung cancer in New Zealand was considerably less than that of the United Kingdom, although New Zealanders are among the heaviest cigarette smokers anywhere.[49] He also found that the death rate of male British immigrants was about twice that of the white native-born males of similar age. Pybus comments that 'the inevitable conclusion was that the British immigrants had brought the seeds of the disease with them; in other words they had come from a highly industrialized country with a heavy air pollution and in consequence had accumulated enough soot or benzpyrene in their lungs to give them this higher mortality.'

Dean carried out a similar study in South Africa confirming the results found in New Zealand.[50] The mortality from lung cancer was less than in the United Kingdom, and in certain age limits the death rate from lung cancer amongst the British immigrants was double that of the native-born white South African males and similar immigrants from other countries, although South Africans are among the heaviest cigarette smokers in the world.

Pybus concludes his discussion of the evidence by saying that 'of all the possible causes of cancer in man, there seems no doubt that the main one is, as far as this country is concerned, smoke from various sources and in different forms. There are many other known cancer producing substances but most play a very small, if any, part in producing the disease. In other countries, other factors, diet, etc may be concerned.'

It is interesting that this conclusion was anticipated many years ago by Evelyn in his *Fumifugium*: 'But in the meantime being thus incorporated with the very Aer, which ministers to the necessary respiration of our Lungs, the Inhabitants of London, and such as frequent it, find it in all their Expectorations; the Spittle, and other excrements which proceed from them, being for the most part of a blackish and fuliginous Colour; Besides this, acrimonious Soot produces another sad effect, by rendering the people obnoxious to Inflammations, and comes (in time) to exulcerate the Lungs, which is a mischief so incurable, that it carries away multitudes by languishing and deep Consumptions, as the Bills of Mortality do Weekly inform us.'[51]

Benzpyrene and other hydrocarbons are not the only agents in industrial and cigarette smoke which may be implicated in the causation of lung cancer. It is known, for instance, that tobacco contains radioactive substances but until recently these were not considered important because their contribution was thought to be very small compared with the radioactivity inhaled from the air. However, early estimates of radioactivity inhaled from the air do not take into account that much of it may be expired before it decays. Radon, for instance, has a half life of 3·8 days. Marsden and Collins [52] have recently calculated that radiation received from the radon in the air would only amount to 0·5 picocuries compared with a previous estimate of 2,000 pc. This is likely to be brought up to about 10 pc by the inclusion of products likely to be produced by radon and the absorption of these on dust particles. This estimate may be compared with one of about 16 pc due to smoking 50 cigarettes a day. It is interesting that increasing use is made of some of the tobaccos which appeared to have a particularly high radioactivity. Marsden and Collins point out that there seems to be a general correspondence between lung cancer statistics and the import figures for these tobaccos.

More recently Marsden[53] has directed attention to a radioactive isotope of polonium which emits alpha particles, believed to be particularly active in initiating changes in protein structure. This polonium-201 may enter the body through tobacco smoke and from car exhaust fumes and moves to the soft tissues of the body such as the lung and the reproductive organs. Again it is interesting to note that the alpha activity of tobacco leaf varies by as much as 30 to 1 according to the type of soil in which the plant is grown, the most active tobaccos being those grown in the most acidic soils. There is also a correspondence between these active tobaccos and the increase of death from lung cancer although the lag is only about ten years rather than the twenty usually thought to elapse.[54]

As additional evidence Marsden points to the fact that the Maoris have a large intake of polonium because they eat great quantities of shell fish which in turn feeds on polonium-rich plankton. Maoris are known to have an especially high incidence of stomach ulcers and it is suggested that this may be caused by their ingestion of polonium. It is interesting to note that polonium is also contained in a lead which is used in antiknock compounds; as this is volatile it escapes into the atmosphere while less volatile lead forms a deposit on car exhaust pipes. If these suggestions are correct, therefore, air pollution is again indicted at least as much as smoking. It hardly needs emphasizing that the source of air pollution here considered, i.e. car exhaust fumes, is an inevitable accompaniment of urbanization.

We are obviously far removed from the very simple kind of hypothesis which we started out with, to wit, 'smoking causes cancer'. We have several causal agents of which smoking may be one; and because smoking has been shown not to be a sufficient cause we must also have factors inside the organism, probably of a constitutional nature, which may interact with these causal factors. The position as it emerges from our discussion is shown in Figure 29. Several possible carcinogenic agents such as urbanization, smoking, air pollution impinge on to an organism which constitutionally is predisposed to react or not to react to these agents with the development of lung cancer. Provided we can identify the causal agents and provided we can identify the constitutional factors in the organism which are responsible for the reaction of the organism to the agent, we should be in a better position to do something constructive about the evil that is lung cancer. It is sometimes said that reference to constitutional factors and to heredity is simply therapeutic nihilism and that once hereditary predisposition is blamed for the reaction of an organism to certain disease producing agencies nothing further can be done. This, however, is quite untrue; once the facts are known something can usually be done and with much better hope of success than if the facts were not known.

As an example of what I have in mind consider the well-known disease called phenylcatonuria which affects about one child in 40,000 in England. Phenylcatonuria causes mental defect and it has been found that about 1 in every 100 patients in hospitals for severely handicapped children, suffers from this disease. The disorder is known to be inherited and children suffering from it can be distinguished from other mentally handicapped or from normal children by testing their urine which yields a green coloured reaction with a solution of ferri-chloride due to the presence of derivatives of phenylalanine. Phenylcatonuria is a perfect example of a disorder produced entirely by hereditary causes where the cause is simple and

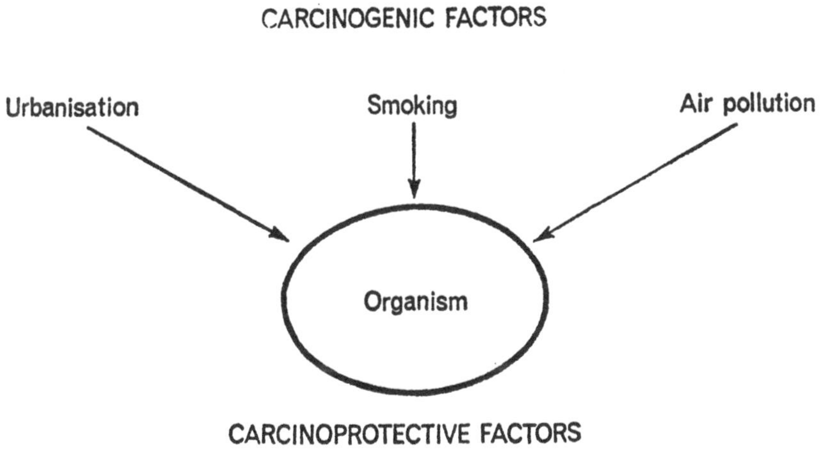

Fig. 29. Diagram illustrating the combined effect on the production of lung cancer of carcinogenic factors such as urbanization, smoking and air pollution and the carcino-protective factors inside the organism which appear to be associated with introverted behaviour, leptosomatic physique, emotionality, etc.

well understood and where the presence of the disorder can be determined with accuracy.

What precisely is it that is inherited? It has been shown that children affected by phenylcatonuria are unable to convert phenylalanine into tyrosine. It is not clear why this should produce mental deficiency but it seems likely that some of the incomplete breakdown products of phenylalanine are poisonous to the nervous system. Now provided that tyrosine is present in the diet phenylalanine fortunately is not an essential part of the food requirements of the child. It is possible to maintain these children on a diet which is almost free of phenylalanine thus eliminating the danger of poisoning to the nervous system. When this method of treatment is begun in the first few months of life there is a very good chance that the child might grow up without the mental handicap he would otherwise have encountered. By thus understanding the precise way in which heredity works we can arrange a rational method of therapy which makes use of the forces of nature rather than trying to counteract them. A realization of the importance of constitutional factors is, of course, only a beginning; what is required is detailed experimental research work which alone can tell us precisely how heredity works in each instance and precisely what it does.

Much research obviously remains to be done in this field. Constitutional factors suggested in the last chapter need to be established on a much firmer basis before we can really feel that we are nearer the heart of the puzzle. It is sad to think, for instance, that there are seven prospective studies on the relationship between smoking and lung cancer in progress, none of which is making use of personality questionnaires to investigate more closely the relationships between both smoking and cancer on the one hand, and extraversion and neuroticism on the other. Many other types of investigations spring to mind which might be useful in throwing light on our problem. We need to know far more about the physiological and biochemical factors in human beings which are related to extraversion and to neuroticism; there are no insoluble problems here in principle. The investigations could make use of well-tried existing methods. Breeding studies in rats along the lines of the emotionality studies mentioned in a previous chapter would also seem to be in order; it has now been established that similar strain differences can be established through breeding with respect to cortical excitation and inhibition, or 'extraversion' and 'introversion' if these terms can meaningfully be applied to rats; here again physiological and neurological studies as well as investigations of hormonal secretions could throw a flood of light on the precise biological basis of these personality dimensions. In this way we might hope to be able to single out the 1 person in 20 who constitutionally is predisposed to interact with cigarette smoking and develops cancer, thus making it possible for the other 19 to enjoy their pleasures without having this dreadful threat hanging over them. What we need clearly is some kind of index as clear as the green urine of the phenylcatonuric child to indicate which persons are at risk.

Must we then after all accept the view that smoking is in part responsible for the development of lung cancer? The data we have reviewed do not give a certain answer to this question, as we have already noted, and they are subject to many serious criticisms. Indeed, the difficulties presented by a problem which contains several hypothetical causal factors and several constitutional interacting factors are such that it may seem impossible to resolve these difficulties by purely statistical means. Fortunately, some accidental events appear to have come to our aid to enable us to come to a more definite conclusion in this matter. Curiously enough the studies to which I am referring now are not even mentioned in either the American or the British reports on smoking and health, nor are they referred to in the otherwise very full treatment given to the subject by C. van Proosdij in his book, *Smoking*. The matter was raised by Dr Jan Beffinger who was born in Poland and who organized on behalf of the Polish Tobacco Monopoly various tobacco plantations and invented and introduced a new method of fermentation of tobacco which was adopted by the USSR Tobacco Industry after the seizure of Poland. Beffinger himself escaped, became British by naturalization, worked for a while in Cyprus and saw military service in the Middle East; since then he has been supervisor of the Tobacco Leaf Production and Cigarette Manufacture in Eritrea, advisor on tobacco to the Ethiopian Tobacco Régime at Addis Abbaba, and is now resident in Kenya.

Dr Beffinger starts out with a fact which is in itself rather startling. If the reader will turn back to Figure 6 which gives the relationship between deaths by lung cancer and cigarette consumption he will find there no mention of countries behind the iron curtain or of South Africa. This is curious because, as Beffinger states: 'It is a statistical fact that in some countries like the Soviet Union, Poland and the Union of South Africa there is no increase in the rate of lung cancer to the same extent as in the USA and the UK – although in those countries the consumption of cigarettes is increasing at the same rate as in the USA and the UK.' Referring to Poland Beffinger points out that 'Yearly figures on lung cancer cases are astonishingly small and hardly change from year to year. Which indicates that they are within the limits of natural causes.' The number of deaths from lung cancer in Poland in 1956, for instance, was less than half that in the UK or the USA. Regarding Russian investigations on tobacco smoking and lung cancer it has been reported by Dr A. B. Savittski of the USSR Academy of Medical Sciences that studies in Russia indicated that there was no relationship between the smoking of cigarettes and lung cancer. 'Russians do not deny that they have cases of lung cancer, especially in industrial areas, but they clearly state that they are not facing the problem to such a catastrophic extent as the UK and the USA.' These facts when taken in conjunction are puzzling and interesting, and demand an explanation. Dr Beffinger is ready with such an explanation.

His argument begins by pointing out that up to the beginning of this century practically all countries were using similar methods of processing their tobacco leaves. This method made use of natural enzymatic fermentation, and the presence of free access of airborne oxygen. However, about 1905 a redrying procedure was introduced in the USA and later in the UK. During this process the tobacco leaf is treated with high temperatures of about 80°C; these high temperatures cause the enzymes to be destroyed and afterwards no enzymatic fermentation of leaf can take place, especially when the leaf is pressed into airtight hogsheads. This procedure lasts only about 45 to 90 minutes as against 3 to 4 months in the case of natural enzymatic fermentation, and the loss of dry weight of leaf processed is only about 2 per cent or less against 12 per cent during natural enzymatic fermentation.

This redrying procedure was not adopted by Soviet Russia, Poland or South Africa, and the cigarettes which were smoked there were exclusively made from tobacco leaves which were fully enzymatically fermented. Beffinger, therefore, suggests that what is responsible for the great differences between the countries listed in our Figure 6, and Russia, Poland and South Africa on the other, is the method of fermentation used for the cigarettes smoked in these countries.

Beffinger goes on to point out that the enzymatic fermentation process gives rise to *alkaline* tobaccos whereas the newer redrying method gives rise to *acid*-type tobaccos, and he also points out that cigars which have been shown not to be connected with lung cancer are essentially produced by methods similar to the old and to give rise to alkaline smoke. In addition Beffinger quotes some experimental work in which it has been shown that alkaline smoke when dissolved in water releases no tar even after several months whereas dissolved acidic smoke yields a tar deposit after only a few hours. In view of the suspicion that has been raised regarding the causal effect of tar on lung cancer this may be an important finding.

Beffinger adduces other rather interesting facts to support his thesis. Thus he points out that the first signs of alarm regarding the increasing rate of lung cancer among cigarette smokers in the United States was raised in the years between 1930 and 1935. 'It is striking that if one takes into consideration that it takes about 25 years for lung cancer to develop in the cigarette smoker that puts the time back to around 1905 which date coincides with the introduction of the tobacco redrying procedure in the USA.'

South Africa is of particular interest in this connection because until quite recently the natural method of enzymatic fermentation was used. 'Then in about 1930 the flue-curing tobacco was introduced and it was followed in 1940 by the introduction of the 're-drying' procedure. Consequently the majority of cigarettes smoked in South Africa from about 1930–40 started to acquire a strongly acid smoke, and 20 to 25 years later in about 1950 the lung cancer incidence in South Africa started to increase and in fact had doubled in a decade; from 1947 to 1956 in comparison to about 25 previous years the cigarette consumption by white South Africans (1922 to 1931) had increased by 36 per cent . . . under the circumstances it should now be expected that due to smoking cigarettes with acid smoke the present lung cancer incidence in South Africa will further increase and will reach the alarming level of the United Kingdom in about 1965–70.' This in brief is the hypothesis put forward by Dr Beffinger and if true it clearly provides considerable evidence in favour of the causal effect of smoking on lung cancer. If it could indeed be shown that people smoking one type of cigarette die of lung cancer much more frequently than people smoking a different kind of cigarette, then this would seem to establish the causal theory once and for all. At the same time of course it would give us a method of counteracting the evil effects of smoking by simply switching from one process of fermentation to another.

The data which Beffinger adduces to support his case are certainly very striking, but again they cannot be said to be conclusive. Like most *post hoc* studies and investigations there are many loopholes here which would need to be filled before the results could be accepted as conclusive. However, given the existence of these two types of cigarettes, i.e. those with an acid and those with an alkaline smoke, it should not be impossible to arrange for a conclusive comparative study. What would be required would be the comparison over a period of years of the death rates from lung cancer of people habitually smoking these two types of cigarettes. Such an experiment ought certainly to be tried because it seems to be the one way in which we can either prove or disprove conclusively the causal hypothesis and also obtain evidence regarding methods of reducing the incidence of lung cancer without having to give up smoking. The neglect of Beffinger's hypothesis by the authorities is curious and it is to be hoped that others will take up his suggestions and carry out the requisite research.

One of the things, therefore, and one of the most urgent that we should do about smoking, is to initiate new research, research that does not simply duplicate what has already been done but that makes use of new theories, new views, new information, in a field where finance has always been the great problem. It seems a trifle absurd that there should be 25 retrospective and 7 prospective studies into the connection between smoking and lung cancer, all of them suffering from the drawbacks in designs and execution we have already discussed and all of them liable to give very similar results. One single well planned and well executed study, or perhaps at most two or three, would seem to be quite sufficient to give us all the information that can be obtained in this manner and by this type of investigation. Such duplication of research effort becomes even harder to understand when it is realized that no efforts are being made to study the influence of constitutional factors or to investigate the importance of different methods of fermentation. More experimentation, and particularly more creatively planned experimentation, based on new theories such as the ones reviewed in this book seem to be called for. Without such new information we are never going to get beyond the present clearly unsatisfactory situation.

Chapter 8

Giving up Smoking?

A cigarette is the perfect type of a perfect pleasure. It is exquisite, and it leaves one unsatisfied. What more can one want?

OSCAR WILDE

THE PRESENT SITUATION is so unsatisfactory because the two main theories, the direct causal theory and the constitutional one, are usually capable of explaining the observed fact equally well so that these facts do not serve to make a choice between them possible. Consider for instance the facts regarding the Seventh Day Adventists in the United States. This sect, which is a non-smoking, non-drinking community, also differs from the general population by having a lower intake of meat, coffee and tea and a higher intake of milk, and appears to be remarkably free from lung cancer.[55] Wynder and Lemon who instigated this study suggested that the results supported a direct causal connection between smoking and lung cancer, but again it must be said that the results can equally well be explained by reference to a constitutional hypothesis. Religious groups like the Seventh Day Adventists tend to be extremely introverted in their personality, and therefore be predisposed constitutionally not to develop lung cancer and not to smoke. Until we are able to leave this vicious circle of alternative hypotheses giving similar predictions clearly we shall not advance very far.

Some people propose to cut the Gordian Knot by direct assertion. The authors of the British and American reports claim that: 'Cigarette smoking is causally related to lung cancer in men; the magnitude of the effect of cigarette smoking far outweighs all other factors.' The data are certainly compatible with such a conclusion, but do they really reinforce it strongly enough to make possible a definite statement of this kind? Can we be certain that there is a causal relationship of this kind in spite of all the weaknesses in the evidence which we have pointed out? The answer to this question lies probably in the ambiguity of the term 'certainty'. It is agreed among philosophers of science and scientists themselves that the scientific, inductive method can never lead to certain conclusions; all scientific endeavour is asymptotic to truth. Historically even the most certain conclusions in science have usually been overthrown within 100 years or so, and others have taken their place. Newton's theory of the corpuscular nature of light became a dogma to such an extent that Dr Thomas Young hardly dared publish his theories regarding the wave theory of light for fear that his patients would cease to regard him as a reliable physician. Yet within 50 years the corpuscular theory had been completely overthrown and the wave theory had become the reigning dogma. By the turn of this cenntry again both theories were seen to be partly right and partly wrong and we now have a combined theory according to which light partakes of the nature of both corpuscles and waves. This way of looking at scientific theories is not one which recommends itself to the layman, and it is not one which the busy physician is likely to look upon with great enthusiasm. Nevertheless, it is the only correct way for the scientist to approach any kind of decision. From this point of view we must say that the case has not been established beyond any doubt. The evidence in favour of the hypothesis that smoking causes cancer is certainly very strong indeed but it is equally certainly not conclusive.

The view is often contested by physicians who argue as follows. 'The evidence that is available to us,' they say 'is not perfect, but it is very strong – so strong that it would go against our conscience as responsible doctors, whose main duty it is to save life, not to warn the population of the risks which they run if they continue to smoke. Ivory tower science no doubt knows no certainty but we live in an imperfect world and we have to make decisions every day on the basis of what we know here and now. When the evidence is so strongly in support of a particular conclusion, and if action can be taken on that conclusion that is likely to save thousands of lives, then surely it would be irresponsible on our part not to suggest taking that action. The eternal search for scientific truth is certainly an admirable adventure of the human spirit, but equally admirable surely is the eternal desire of the physician to save life.'

Some physicians even go further than that. They claim that to publish critical surveys of the evidence (like the present one) is in fact irresponsible because it lowers the belief of readers in the general conclusion which they support, namely that smoking causes cancer, and may therefore lead some people into deciding that giving up smoking may not be as necessary as they had thought on reading the medical reports. On this view what is needed is a large scale propaganda campaign to bring home to every man, woman and child the dangers involved in smoking, and all voices that would speak out against this view are therefore doing a disservice to society.

This conflict between the clinical and the scientific way of looking at things is, of course, a very old one, and has received some interesting experimental illumination at the hands of some American psychologists. What was done was to get together a large number of experimentalists and a large number of clinicians, and then to administer to each of these in turn a test. The test consisted simply of the old 'pea under the thimble' trick, known to most frequenters of race courses. The subject is shown three thimbles on a board; he is also shown a pea. The experimenter puts the pea under one of the thimbles then shuffles the three thimbles about and asks the subject to say under which thimble the pea is located. After the choice is made the thimble indicated is lifted up and the subject finds that he has been mistaken. The thimbles are moved around again and the subject makes another choice. Again he is mistaken. So the game continues until finally, after a large number of consecutive failures, the subject voices a suspicion that the experimenter has in fact removed the pea by a trick so that he cannot win under any conditions.

Now, of course, there is no certainty attending this conclusion on the part of the experimentalists or clinicians, but it is interesting to see that in fact the clinicians arrive at this conclusion very much earlier than did the experimentalists who required many more trials before voicing their suspicions. In other words, certainty, as the term is used in ordinary human discourse, is a psychological quality attaching to certain phenomena, and there are great individual differences in our perception of this particular quality. Some people would regard it as certain that the pea had been removed if they failed 10 or 12 times running; others would go on for 500 or even 1,000 trials before they arrived at an equal state of certainty. Now it must be noted that there is nothing right or wrong about this; these are psychological peculiarities of people which govern their actions, and all that one can say is that the person who has a low level of certainty, as it were, will be likely to be wrong far more often than the person who has a high level of certainty. On the other hand, of course, the person who requires a high level of certainty may waste a good deal of his time repeating experiences in order to make assurance doubly sure. This difference in temperament is probably itself connected with extraverted and introverted behaviour patterns; extraverts are quick to form conclusions, introverts are much slower. It is also known that scientists tend to be introverted, physicians and other clinicians extraverted. Thus what may appear at first sight as a philosophical or scientific dispute is at bottom perhaps nothing more than a clash of different types of temperament.[56]

The question still remains. Should the scientist for the sake of possibly saving a large number of lives keep his doubts quiet or only voice them in scientific publications? It is often assumed that propaganda campaigns such as those based on the two medical reports on smoking and health do in fact put people off smoking. Berkson has thrown some doubt on this matter. This is what he has to say.[57] 'What has happened to the per capita consumption of cigarettes since this furore of smoking causing lung cancer was launched? As is shown [in Figure 30] the per capita consumption per annum was going down till 1954 – when

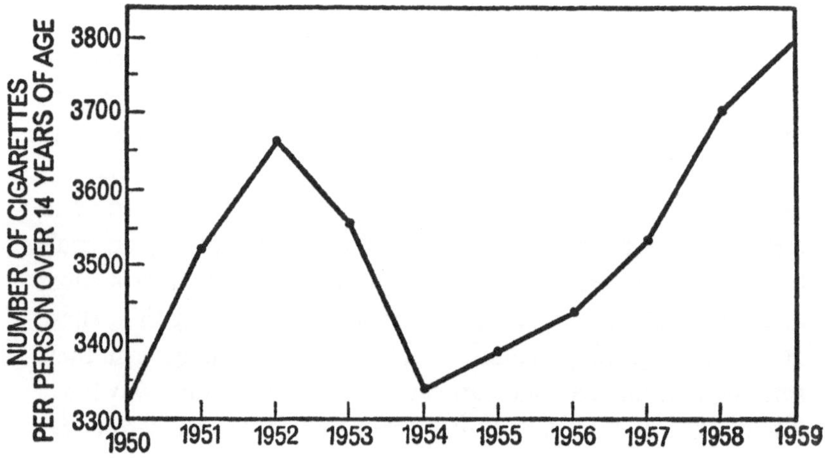

Fig. 30. Per capita consumption per annum of cigarettes. The speedy descent in consumption beginning in 1952 was converted by a rapid rise beginning in 1955, just after the reports identifying smoking as the chief cause of lung cancer were announced. In 1959 it stood well above its previous maximum. The data are for the United States and the figure is reproduced with permission from J. Berkson, *American Statistican*, 1963, 17, 19.

these investigations were announced. Then it turned and began rising precipitously. The last year for which I plotted it, 1959, shows the highest consumption ever attained up to that time. According to preliminary reports 1963 will surpass even that. I will not insist that this is an association of cause and effect; but it is fairly probable. The American public has been made cigarette conscious by this discussion as they have never been before, and cigarette sales have mounted. The tobacco industry and those who own tobacco stock of whom unhappily I am not one have benefited, but has anyone else? The whole discussion has been conducted in an atmosphere of emotion and recrimination. We ought to cool it off and engage in some sober and responsible thought on all aspects of the problem, and particularly the research aspects.'

Evidence in other countries has shown a variety of reactions to the publication of these reports. Usually there has been an immediate fall but a gradual or not so gradual return to pre-report levels and beyond. It is doubtful if on the whole the reports have had much of an effect on the public, with the possible exception of doctors who seem to have stopped smoking to a significant extent. All this is perhaps not too difficult to understand. Berkson added that: 'If a campaign is undertaken it would be well to consult sociologists and psychologists as to how the campaign should be conducted lest it have more bad effect than good.' Social psychologists have shown only too clearly that propaganda campaigns of whatever kind and however good the intention behind them, may have effects quite different to those anticipated. Consider for instance, some studies carried out by the American Army during the Second World War. The aim of these investigations was to find out what kind of propaganda film would be best suited to convince soldiers that the war in Japan would soon be over. The experiment I want to discuss was essentially concerned with a very simple question. Would the film be more effective if it concentrated entirely on putting the one side, or would it be more effective if it stressed the conclusion that the war would soon be over, but also gave some arguments in the other direction, if only to quash them finally? Audiences exposed to these films were pretested and grouped according to their intelligence into bright and dull, and also according to their present expectation of the length of the war in Japan into those whose views were in accordance with the propaganda aims of the film and those whose views were discordant. It was found that dull people whose views were discordant were persuaded by the single sided presentation and changed their views in line with the expressed purpose of the film. However, dull people whose views were in accordance with the aims of the film and who saw the one that presented both sides were actually moved away from the desired conclusion into believing that the war would last longer than they thought to begin with! Intelligent people generally reacted poorly to the film that gave only one side, and for those who had originally believed that the war would soon be over the effect was actually in the opposite direction; the one-sidedness of the film presumably made them suspicious! In other words, there are great complexities in this field and the idea that simply publishing medical reports or brief newspaper articles about these reports would have very much of an effect on the smoking habits of people is not a tenable one.

The whole problem is a particularly difficult one because of the well-known *law of temporal succession.* This law, put quite briefly and baldly, states that if an act has two consequences, one rewarding and the other punishing, which would be strictly equal if simultaneous, then the influence of those consequences upon later performances of the act will vary depending upon the order in which they occur. If the punishing consequences comes first and the rewarding one later the difference between the inhibiting and the reinforcing effect will be in favour of the inhibition, but if the rewarding consequence comes first and the punishing one later the difference will be in favour of the reinforcement.[58] This formulation of the law was made by O. H. Mowrer who comments as follows: 'One can think of this problem in terms of a physical analogy. If two weights of equal mass are placed at equal distances from the fulcrum of a lever they will, of course, exactly counterbalance each other; but if either of these objectively 'equal' weights is placed further from the fulcrum than the other it has a mechanical advantage which enables it to tip the balance in its favour. In the functional sense the weights are no longer 'equal' and a state of 'disbalance' results. In this physical analogy *spatial distance* from the fulcrum provides the advantage whereas in the psychological situation it is *temporal nearness* to the rewarding or punishing state of affairs that is the deciding factor. In this sense the analogy is not an entirely happy one but it will suffice to illustrate the point that in a dynamic (conflict) situation the outcome is determined not only by the absolute magnitude of the causal forces but also by their relational properties.'

If we apply this law to the smoking of cigarettes we can see how very strongly it works against the giving up of smoking. The reward is immediate; the punishing consequences are not only very problematical but they are also in the far distance. No wonder then that although some people give up smoking when they first read about the dangers involved, they will soon drift back into it, and that others will not even bother to give it up at all. Something much more positive would be called for than the propaganda effects of medical reports of this kind if we want to counteract the law of temporal succession.

This argument assumes, of course, that people do not act in a rational manner, but that their actions are governed completely by some form of hedonistic law. This view is often disputed by theologians and others who believe in 'free will', but the notion of free will and rational choice does not receive very much support from an unbiased view of human activities. Even if we take a purely rational point of view, however, we might not perhaps come to the anticipated conclusion. Let us consider the case of a man who is smoking heavily, derives great enjoyment and support from it, and who is faced with the kind of arguments we have presented throughout this book. Is it rational for him to give up smoking or continue to do so? If he continues smoking heavily then he runs the risk of having at the end of 75 a shorter life than a non-smoker by roughly 1·4 years. He might reasonably reply that there are so many hazards involved in life in any case that this relatively short period of longer life, problematical as it is, would certainly not compensate him for the lack of pleasure which would be involved in giving up smoking. Is this a rational or an irrational attitude?

The answer depends of course very much on the person involved, his values, his history and many other factors which are quite individual to each person; it is impossible to come to any general conclusion. Certainly many people when questioned give some such answer in explanation of why they don't give up smoking; the immediate loss of pleasure and satisfaction is not compensated for by the problematical increase of a year or two in their life span at the age of 70 or above.

Even if people do make the decision that they ought to give up smoking it is well known that the law of temporal succession makes this extremely difficult for them. The pleasure following the smoking is immediate; the satisfaction following the giving up of smoking is long delayed and never as clear-cut and definite. No wonder that there are great difficulties in the way of giving up smoking, and that no foolproof method has yet been discovered. The best way is probably a combination of two methods using both the physiological effects of nicotine and the psychological methods of negative practice or conditioned inhibition as it is sometimes called.[59] The physiological part of the treatment consists essentially in the giving of small doses of nicotine in tablet form; many people get a definite 'lift' from smoking a cigarette which comes from the pharmacologically stimulant activity of nicotine. This can also be obtained from tablets of lobeline which is a drug pharmacologically strongly resembling nicotine and which does not seem to be an addictive drug.

One way in which nicotine may provide this lift is by stimulating the smoker's adrenal gland to excrete a hormone (epinephrine) which in turn stimulates the production of glycogen (blood sugar) thus giving the smoker renewed energy. It has been suggested that this rise in blood sugar is a source of a considerable part of the gratification produced by smoking; this effect would, of course, be additional to the stimulant effect on the cortex which we had noted before. The theory of the use of lobeline would be that it provides this lift and would thus be used instead of a cigarette. G. Edwards (*Medical Officer*, 1964,

112, 158–60) recently checked the claims made for this drug by comparing two groups of patients, one of whom was given lobeline tablets, the other dummy tablets which had no pharmacological effect of any kind. He found that 'Neither during the 4-week treatment nor at follow-up were there significant differences in outcome between the two groups.' It is clear that drug treatment of this type by itself is not very useful and most experts in the field agree that it must be joined with some form of psychological treatment.

The psychological side, however, presents much greater difficulties and many 'tricks' and psychological cures have been suggested by a variety of writers. Proosdij in his excellent book on smoking comments that 'Like the editors of the *British Medical Journal*, one could maintain that all these "smoking cures" are fruitless if resoluteness, the only indispensable quality, is lacking.' Statements such as these are of course psychologically somewhat meaningless. People do not have a quality of 'resoluteness', or a definite quantity of 'will-power' which they can bring to bear on this or any other problem. Indeed, the only evidence for this alleged will-power leading to the giving up of a habit is the very giving up of the habit which the concept of will-power or resoluteness is supposed to explain. Pseudo-psychological notions of this type which are often advanced by non-psychologists are not very helpful and merely cloud the issue. They may even do harm; many people who wish to give up smoking state that they have no 'will-power' and therefore refrain from even making the effort. What then can be done?

The answer will I am afraid sound very mechanistic to most readers.[60] Essentially it depends again on the law of temporal succession. In the ordinary way people find it difficult to give up smoking because the reward (or more technically, 'reinforcement') is immediate for any violation of the no-smoking rule, and thus a very strong habit is being reinforced every time the rule is broken. Rewarding consequences on the other hand are remote and ill-defined. In order to alter this situation what we must do quite obviously is to have punishing consequences follow the smoking of a cigarette *before* the rewarding consequences have any chance to establish themselves. This is the method suggested by Dr G. J. S. Wilde from Amsterdam. Dr Wilde has constructed an apparatus which consists essentially of a ventilator heater into which can be introduced 10 lighted cigarettes which are then 'smoked' by the ventilator and whose smoke comes out, diffused in the hot air produced by the ventilator. This mixture of hot air is extremely unpleasant and, of course, it resembles in many respects the effect of smoking. This Wilde calls the *aversive stimulus.* He also has a second ventilator which produces a somewhat slower stream of air at room temperature (without heat or smoke) in which a little bit of menthol from an aerosol is diffused; this he calls the reward, and it is experienced as being very agreeable and refreshing. When the reward stimulus is presented the subject is also permitted to take a small peppermint from a dish whenever he likes; this is a substitute behaviour for smoking, which the subject intends to learn.

During the treatment sessions the smoker is asked to light a cigarette of his preferred brand. Simultaneously the aversive stimulus is administered i.e. the hot air full of cigarette smoke is blown straight at him. The smoker has to keep the cigarette in his mouth until he cannot tolerate the aversive stimulus in combination with his own cigarette any longer. As soon as he puts the cigarette out and pronounces the auto-suggestive phrase 'I want to give up smoking' the rewarding stimulus is administered and he is allowed to take a peppermint if he wishes. The trials are repeated a number of times depending on the subject's report of his tolerance, varying from 6 to 20 times in succession. Then the aversive stimulus is cut out and the smoker is invited to light a cigarette without the aversive stimulus. This is done in order to have him feel that the cigarette itself has become offensive and sickening. This cigarette is usually put out as quickly as the ones during aversive stimulation, that is after 2 to 3 pulls. This session is then ended with some instructions to the smoker under treatment which have to be followed until the next session 24 hours later. These instructions are: 'If you happen to feel like a cigarette try to remember the treatment session, try to experience the sensation of relief when putting out the cigarette and saying that you want to give up smoking; take a peppermint or something similar instead. If you give in nevertheless keep the cigarette in your mouth until you cannot stand it any more and extinguish it.'

This method capitalizes on the law of temporal succession by making the consequences of smoking exceedingly unpleasant. Furthermore this unpleasantness follows immediately upon the lighting of the cigarette and consequently has a maximum chance of setting up a conditioned aversive response. This psychological treatment, combined with lobeline in cases where a physical need appears to have been established, should suffice to reinforce the hypothetical 'will-power' of even the most average and ordinary person to a sufficient extent to enable him to give up smoking. It is likely that one or two booster doses of the treatment may be required, but this should not give rise to any undue difficulties in extinguishing the undesired habit. To those who are familiar with modern behaviouristic methods of treating neurotic disorders and other undesirable habit patterns [61] it will be obvious that there are other possible ways of extinguishing this particular habit; I have stressed the one developed by Wilde because his method is the only one that has been applied in practice and been shown to be useful. Here, too, it must be added that much further research will be necessary, particularly on the interaction between method of treatment and personality of smoker, before we can say that we have come to any final solution of the problem.

This indeed is the main message that this book has to carry. What is needed is more fundamental research rather than more dogmatic statements. It may be true that where there is smoke there is fire, but it is also obvious that very little has been positively achieved to date. What we think we know is largely surmised, and even if most of it were true it would not help us to take any practical steps to overcome the menace of lung cancer and coronary disease. Epidemiological methods of investigation have set up a problem; they have not handed us a solution. That solution must await more determined experimental efforts.

Epilogue

Where there's Smoke there's Fire

Non fumum ex fulgore, sed ex fumo dare lucem cogitat.

HORACE

WE STARTED OUT with the question: Does smoking cause cancer? Prosecution and defence have both had their say; what is the verdict? Clearly the accused does not emerge with an untarnished reputation. Studies of the lungs of smokers and non-smokers reveal deleterious after-effects very clearly among the former; dangerous substances are precipitated in the lungs, and the ciliary movements by means of which these substances are normally removed are themselves impeded by smoke. Some of these substances, such as the cyclic hydrocarbons and some radioactive isotopes of polonium, are known to or suspected of producing cancerous growths. Clearly, smoking is not likely to promote anyone's health, and suspicion is very strong that cigarette smoking may indeed be a killer. However, in science as in law, the accused is presumed innocent unless proven guilty, and it must be said that the evidence, although strong, is not conclusive; it is circumstantial rather than direct, and it does not demonstrate the case against smoking 'beyond any reasonable doubt'. This conclusion of 'not proven' must, of course, leave open the question of just how reasonable doubt is at this juncture; we have pointed out that scientific evidence is never 'certain' in the philosophical meaning of that term, and that different people have different psychological thresholds of 'certainty' which will determine what they are prepared to regard as 'reasonable' in the way of doubt.

If the evidence appears strong in pointing to a statistical correlation between smoking and lung cancer, then it must be added that the actual numerical values often cited are subject to so many errors and inaccuracies that they should be regarded with the greatest caution. The populations studied have clearly not been representative; the refusal rate among those asked to take part in these investigations has been much too large for comfort; and the ascertainment of smoking habits has been subject both to errors of memory and of estimation. Little attention has been paid to different ways of smoking, such as number of pulls taken, length of pull, and length of stub thrown away; all of these may powerfully affect the numerical estimates. Worst of all, the smokers and non-smokers studied have been self-selected, thus allowing alternative hypotheses to be put forward to explain the statistical correlations. Experimental studies have shown the existence of such self-selective factors, and their importance in producing statistical relationships without any direct causal implication.

An alternative hypothesis to that of direct causal relation between smoking and lung cancer has been put forward, postulating that the statistical results obtained may be due to the fact that persons constitutionally predisposed to take up smoking are also constitutionally predisposed to develop cancer. Evidence has been brought forward to show that persons of an extraverted temperament are both more likely to smoke cigarettes, and to develop cancer, than are persons of an introverted temperament. While this evidence is not based on sufficient numbers of cases to establish the point definitively, it must be said that the congruence between several studies which has been a notable point of our survey lends some credence to the hypothesis. A further point in its favour is the established relationship between smoking, cancer proneness, and pyknic (squat, stocky) body build; persons of this body type are known to have predominantly extraverted types of temperament.

The hypothesis that cigarette smoking causes cancer is so appealing because it satisfies simultaneously two sets of relations. In the first place it explains the statistical correlation between smoking and cancer; in the second place it explains the rapid growth in the incidence of lung cancer in recent years, which agrees well with the growth of cigarette consumption. The constitutional hypothesis explains the first of these sets of relations; the second is possibly best explained by reference to the growth in air pollution. Urban air contains the same cyclic hydrocarbons and radioactive isotopes as tobacco smoke, and in addition contains them in much greater profusion. This hypothesis would also serve to explain the close correlation between lung cancer rates and degree of urbanization, a correlation which is not due to differences in smoking habits.

This is the factual position at the moment. There are two main hypotheses on the market; both can explain the facts, both have certain difficulties in the evidence to contend with, and both fail to provide that definitive proof which scientists require. Cigarette smoking is neither a necessary nor a sufficient cause of lung cancer; the evidence suggests but does not prove that it is an important contributory cause. The evidence also suggests, however, that atmospheric pollution is probably an even more important factor, and that it would be unwise to concentrate all available research efforts and legislative measures on smoking. It is psychologically much easier to cause people to give up those habits which lead to atmospheric pollution than to give up smoking, and if our aim is the lessening of the terrible toll which lung cancer takes of life nowadays this avenue seems to be the more promising to take. Research into the effects of smoking should certainly be continued, particularly with reference to the possible interaction between smoking, personality and constitution, and the facts unearthed should be communicated to the public. But what is communicated should really be well-established facts, not statistical surmises based on largely unproven and sometimes even improbable assumptions. Most important, research should be directed at the search for direct, causal physiological and neurological variables, rather than for circumstantial evidence supporting purely statistical calculations.

In the end, I believe (although I cannot at the moment prove) that both the hypotheses under discussion will be found to be true. I believe that *in certain people*, and *under certain conditions*, smoking acts in such a manner as to upset the delicate balance between carcinogenic and carcinoprotective factors; it may thus interact with constitutional and environmental conditions in very complex ways to produce its deleterious effects. I believe these effects are less important than suggested by the calculations in the British and the American Reports, and I also believe that atmospheric pollution, acting in a similar manner, is much more important than it has been given credit for. I believe that the most important need at the moment is for research into the problems I have raised in the course of the discussion, but I also believe that definite action should be taken to reduce the danger from air pollution. After all, we choose whether we want to smoke, but we have no choice of whether we want to breathe or not! There is no reason why society should be allowed to poison our lungs, but every reason why we should be allowed to poison our own if we want to. If we do so choose, then I suggest that we smoke cigarettes which are made from tobacco grown in the least acidic soils, and cured by enzymatic fermentation. And to end, I cannot do better than quote again from Evelyn's *Fumifugium*: 'Whilst these are belching it forth their sooty jaws, the City of London resembles the face rather of Mount Etna, the Court of Vulcan, Stromboli, or the Suburbs of Hell, than an Assembly of Rational Creatures, and the Imperial seat of our Incomparable Monarch.

'For when in all other places the Aer is most Serene and Pure, it is here Ecclipsed with such a Cloud of Sulphure, as the Sun itself, which gives day to all the World besides, is hardly able to penetrate and impart it here: and the weary Traveller, at many Miles distance, sooner smells, than sees the City to which he repairs.

'This is that pernicious Smoake which sullyes all her Glory, superinducing a sooty Crust or Fur upon all that it lights, spoyling the moveables, tarnishing the Plate, Gildings and

Furniture, and corroding the very Iron-bars and hardest Stones with those piercing and acrimonious Spirits which accompany its Sulphure; and executing more in one year, than exposed to the pure Aer of the Country, it could effect in some hundreds.

'It is this horrid Smoake which obscures our Churches, and makes our Palaces look old, which fouls our Clothes, and corrupts the Waters, so as the very Rain, and refreshing Dews which fall in the several Seasons, precipitate this impure vapour, which, with its black and tenacious quality, spots and contaminates whatever is exposed to it.

'Let it be considered what a Fuliginous crust is yearly contracted, and adheres to the Sides of our ordinary Chimnies where this grosse Fuell is used; and then imagine, if there were a solid Tentorium or Canopy over London, what a masse of Soote would then stick to it, which now (as was said) comes down every Night in the Streets, on our Houses, and Waters, and is taken into our Bodies.

'And may this much suffice concerning the Causes and Effects of this Evill, and to discover to all the World, how pernicious this Smoake is to our Inhabitants of London to decrie it, and to introduce some happy Expedient, whereby they may for the Future, hope to be freed from so intolerable an inconvenience.'

Notes

1. An excellent introduction to the history of smoking is given by C. van Proosdij in his book *Smoking* (London, Elsenier, 1960). He also gives detailed references.
2. Topley and Wilson's *Principles of Bacteriology and Immunity*, **2**, 1141 (Baltimore, Williams and Wilkins, 1955).
3. A good source of reference for epidemiological methodology is J. Yerushalmy and C. E. Palmer, *J. Chronic Diseases*, 1959, **10**, 27–40.
4. See J. Yerushalmy, 'Statistical considerations and evaluation of epidemiological evidence', in *Tobacco and Health*, Ed. G. James and T. Rosenthal (C. C. Thomas, Springfield, Ill., 1962).
5. L. Kreyberg, *Brit. J. Cancer*, 1961, **15**, 51–3. Also Histological Lung Cancer Types, *Norwegian Monographs on Medical Science*, 1962.
6. More recent American work has thrown some doubt on the clear-cut nature of the distinction made by Kreyberg.
7. Detailed references and discussions are contained in *Smoking and Health*, a report published in 1964 by the US Dept. of Health, Education and Welfare. This will be referred to in this book as the 'American Report'. Since the publication of this report Doll and Hill have published the latest results of their work (*Brit. Med. J.*, 1964, **1**, 3099–1410, 1460–67). Their main conclusions are most elegantly summarized in the two figures given by them. The first shows the increase in death rate from lung cancer with increase in smoking; the second shows the decrease in death rate from lung cancer in men who had continued smoking and those who had given up smoking cigarettes for varying lengths of time. The great regularity of the data increases one's belief in the reality of the association.
8. Note also the omission of countries like the USSR, Poland and South Africa; as we shall see later, they do not fall in line with the countries plotted.
9. For a critical discussion of the statistical issues involved in this

distinction, see J. Berkson and L. Elveback, *J. Amer. Stat. Ass.*, 1960, **55**, 415–28.

10. *Smoking and Health*, a report of the Royal College of Physicians, published in 1962 by Pitman (London) will be referred to as the 'British Report' throughout this book.
11. J. Berkson, *American Statistician*, 1963, **17**, 15–22. A great deal of work has been done on the experimental side in recent years which is not mentioned by Berkson, and which is too technical to be summarized in a book of this kind. A good account will be found in an article by E. L. Wynder and D. Hoffman, *Experimental Tobacco Carcinogenesis, Advances in Cancer Res.*, 1964, Vol. 8, 249–453. While one must agree with Berkson that these studies fail to give completely convincing direct evidence of a relationship, it cannot be denied, I think, that they do strongly support the statistical evidence.
12. J. Berkson, *Proc. Staff Meetings Mayo Clinic*, 1960, **35**, 367–85. Cf. also *J. Amer. Statistical Ass.*, 1958, **53**, 28–38; *Lancet*, 1962, 14th April, 807–8, and *J. Amer. Statistical Ass.*, 1960, **55**, 415–28.
13. H. J. Eysenck, *Psychology of Politics* (Routledge & Kegan Paul, London, 1953).
14. J. Yerushalmy, in *Tobacco and Health*, *op. cit.*
15. This striking study should be repeated; the number of cases involved is too small to make the conclusions acceptable at a high level of statistical significance. I understand that it has recently been repeated, with much larger numbers, and with similar results.
16. J. Yerushalmy, *Amer. J. Obst. & Gyn.*, 1964, **88**, 505–18.
17. J. Berkson, *Amer. J. Public Health*, 1962, **52**, 1318–29.
18. H. J. Eysenck, *Dimensions of Personality* (Routledge & Kegan Paul, London, 1947).
19. See for instance S. Rachman (Ed.), *Critical Essays on Psychoanalysis* (Pergamon Press, Oxford, 1963).
20. See H. J. Eysenck, *The Structure of Human Personality* (Methuen, London, 1960).
21. Routledge & Kegan Paul, London, 1964.
22. Routledge & Kegan Paul, London, 1965.
23. *Monozygotic Twins* (Oxford University Press, 1962).
24. Cf. H. J. Eysenck (Ed.), *Experiments in Personality* (Routledge & Kegan Paul, London, 1960) Vol. 1. The work described was carried out by Dr P. L. Broadhurst.
25. H. J. Eysenck, *The Dynamics of Anxiety and Hysteria* (Routledge & Kegan Paul, London, 1957).
26. H. J. Eysenck (Ed.), *Experiments with Drugs* (Pergamon Press, Oxford, 1963).

27. K. M. Warwick and H. J. Eysenck, *Life Sciences*, 1963, **4**, 219–25.
28. H. J. Eysenck *et al.*, *Brit. Med. J.*, 1960, **1**, 1456–60.
29. It is interesting to note that alcohol used to be employed to deaden pain during surgery and dental treatment prior to the discovery of ether and chloroform!
30. H. J. Eysenck *Personality and cigarette smoking*, *Life Sciences*, 1964, **3**, 777–92.
31. H. J. Eysenck *et al.*, *Brit. Med. J.*, *op. cit.*
32. H. J. Eysenck, *Smoking, personality and psychosomatic disorders*, *J. Psychosm. Res.*, 1963, **7**, 107–30.
33. An excellent and detailed review is given by J. D. Matarazzo and G. Saslow, *Psychol. Bull.*, 1960, **57**, 493–513. See also the American Report, *op. cit.*
34. Cf. chapter by Dr L. Rees in H. J. Eysenck, *Handbook of Abnormal Psychology* (Pitman, London, 1960).
35. A good review of these studies is given in the American Report.
36. A good if somewhat credulous review is given by L. Le Shan, *J. Nat. Cancer Inst.*, 1959, **22**, 1–18.
37. L. Le Shan and R. E. Worthington, *Brit. J. Med. Psychol.*, 1956, **29**, 49–56; *J. nerv. ment. Dis.*, 1956, **124**, 460–65.
38. D. M. Kissen, *Emotional Factors in Pulmonary Tuberculosis* (Tavistock, London, 1958).
39. O. Hagnell, *Svenska Läk.-Tdn.*, 1961, **58**, 492–98.
40. D. M. Kissen and H. J. Eysenck, *J. Psychosomat. Res.*, 1962, *6*, 123–27.
41. *Brit. Med. J.*, 6th July 1963, 18–19.
42. For details of the M.P.I. see the Manual of the test, University of London Press, 1959. A new, improved version, called the E.P.I., is now available.
43. D. M. Kissen, *Lancet*, 1946, 25th January, 216–17. See also the same author, Brit. J. med. Psychol., 1964, **37**, 203–16.
44. In J. J. Groen *et al.*; Het acute myocardinfarct: een psychosomatische studie a (Bohn, Harlem, 1964).
45. S. F. Buck and D. A. Brown, *Tobacco Res. Council Res. Papers* No. 7.
46. F. C. Pybus, *Newcastle Med. J.*, 1963, **28**, 31–66.
47. P. Stocks, *Brit. J. Cancer*, 1960, **14**, 397–408.
48. S. F. Buck and D. A. Brown, *op. cit.* In an even more recent study by A. J. Wicken and S. F. Buck (*Tobacco Research Council, Research Paper No. 8*), the authors concern themselves with air pollution of employment, as well as with the air pollution of different localities of an administrative district, and found that there was an association between level of air pollution and lung

cancer and bronchitis; the differences in level of lung cancer incidence between rural and urban districts in their study too were not fully accounted for by the age, smoking habits and social class characteristics of the areas involved.

49. D. Eastcott, *Lancet*, 1956, **i**, 37–8.
50. G. Dean, *Brit. Med. J.*, 1959, **ii**, 852–54. A different hypothesis to account for Dean's results is proposed by Beffinger, whose views will be considered below. Dean's most latest results are reported in the *Proceedings of the Royal Society of Medicine*, 1964, **57**, 984–87. He concludes again that 'If smoking characteristics and the number of cigarettes smoked had been the only factors contributing to lung cancer, it would not have been unreasonable to expect them to have led to higher lung cancer rates in South Africa than in Britain, instead of vice versa.' He also makes a rather interesting suggestion, which follows from a comparison of the lung cancer mortality rates in the Channel Islands which at each level of smoking are several times the South African rates, and of approximately the same order and magnitude as the estimated rates of England and Wales. He says: 'It is therefore difficult to believe that the damp, cold climate and over-crowded living conditions of Britain and the Channel Islands, with the repeated respiratory infections that result, do not contribute very considerably to the differences between the lung cancer rate of these areas and South Africa.'

    Good summaries of the most recent work are available in a paper by G. W. Griffith (*Progress in Cancer Research*, 1963, 86–94). He concludes that 'two main factors of aetiological significance are currently drawing attention – cigarette smoke and atmospheric pollution. It cannot be claimed, however, that a satisfactory synthesis of ideas has been achieved. In particular the interaction of these two factors is not yet fully elucidated.' It is possible, as W. Haenszel, D. B. Loveland and M. G. Sirken have suggested (*J. Nat. Cancer Inst.*, 1962, **28**, 947), that there are interaction effects between air pollution and cigarette smoking so that the one may potentiate the other.
51. J. Evelyn, *Fumifugium*. Reprinted by the National Smoke Abatement Soc., 1933.
52. E. Marsden and M. A. Collins, *Nature*, 1963, 8th June, 962–64.
53. E. Marsden, *Nature*, 1964, 18th July, 230–33. For a general review of inhaled radioactive particles and gases, see *Nature*, 1964, 25th July, 352–55, and December, 1964, issue of Health Physics.
54. Beffinger has also drawn attention to the importance of avoiding acidic factors in tobacco, although he is more concerned with

fermentation processes than with soil characteristics; his views are considered on pages 133-7

55. E. C. Wynder and F. R. Lemon, *Calif. Med.*, 1958, **89**, 267–75.
56. In statistics this difference between 'Errors of type one' and 'Errors of type two' was introduced by Sir R. Fisher.
57. *Amer. Statistician*, 1963, **17**, 15–22. See also F. Pygott, *Brit. J. Preventive and Soc. Med.* 1964, **18**, No. 3.
58. O. H. Mowrer, *Learning Theory and Personality Dynamics* (Ronald, New York, 1950).
59. H. J. Eysenck, *Behaviour Therapy and the Neuroses* (Pergamon Press, Oxford, 1960). *Experiments in Behaviour Therapy* (Pergamon Press, Oxford, 1964).
60. G. J. S. Wilde, 'Behaviour therapy for addicted cigarette smokers,' *Behav. Res. & Therapy*, 1964, **2**, 107–10.
61. H. J. Eysenck and S. Rachman, *Causes and Cures of Neurosis* (Routledge & Kegan Paul, London, 1964).

Index